D1521936

Organ Donation in Japan

Organ Donation in Japan

A Medical Anthropological Study

Maria-Keiko Yasuoka

LEXINGTON BOOKS
Lanham • Boulder • New York • London

Published by Lexington Books
An imprint of The Rowman & Littlefield Publishing Group, Inc.
4501 Forbes Boulevard, Suite 200, Lanham, Maryland 20706
www.rowman.com

Unit A, Whitacre Mews, 26-34 Stannary Street, London SE11 4AB

Copyright © 2015 by Lexington Books

All rights reserved. No part of this book may be reproduced in any form or by any electronic or mechanical means, including information storage and retrieval systems, without written permission from the publisher, except by a reviewer who may quote passages in a review.

British Library Cataloguing in Publication Information Available

Library of Congress Cataloging-in-Publication Data

Yasuoka, Maria-Keiko.
Organ donation in Japan : a medical anthropological study / Maria-Keiko Yasuoka.
pages cm
Includes bibliographical references and index.
ISBN 978-1-4985-1566-5 (cloth : alk. paper) -- ISBN 978-1-4985-1567-2 (electronic)
1. Donation of organs, tissues, etc.--Japan. 2. Donation of organs, tissues, etc.--Social aspects--Japan.
I. Title.
RD120.63.J3.Y37 2015
362.17'830952--dc23
2015001616

♾ ™ The paper used in this publication meets the minimum requirements of American National Standard for Information Sciences Permanence of Paper for Printed Library Materials, ANSI/NISO Z39.48-1992.

Printed in the United States of America

To the memory of Dr. Terence Lyons and my father.

Contents

List of Figures and Tables

FIGURES

TABLES

Acknowledgments

In completing this book I have been greatly indebted to the extensive work of many scholars, especially in the field of anthropological research involving many informants. All my work, including both my fieldwork and my research for the American Anthropological Association, would have been much more arduous without the help of several people in both the United States and Japan. Although I can't list them all here, I would like especially to thank the following people who have supported me so strongly, including some who very sadly passed away during the period of my research.

Thank you to the medical staff and transplant surgeons of the University of California San Francisco Medical Center, Kinki University Hospital, Osaka University Hospital, Tokyo Women's Medical University Hospitals, and Tsukuba University Hospital: you were extremely helpful. Special thanks are due to Dr. Takahiro Akiyama, Dr. Norihide Fukushima, Dr. Shinichi Nunoda, Dr. Shiro Takahara, Dr. Kazunari Tanabe, and Dr. Kenji Yuzawa—I'm grateful that you agreed to allow me to interview you when I visited your hospitals and devoted your precious time to my research during your busy schedules.

Thank you to the recipients: for all your support, especially when you invited me to your homes or somewhere private in order to be interviewed freely, even when the tears flowed, and after the interviews for welcoming me into your transplanted lives. In spite of my basic questions, you answered me fully, choosing every word carefully to help the world to gain a greater understanding of the daily lives of organ recipients. In addition, I am grateful to recipient candidates in Stanford University Hospital and Mr. Michikata Okubo, Mr. Masanori Suzuki, Mr. Hiroshi Shimono, and Mr. Kenji Oda of the Japan Transplant Recipients Organization.

Thank you to the donor families: I owe special thanks in particular to six donor family members—you helped me by recounting your bitter experiences, even while weeping again at the pain of recalling and narrating your stories of your lost children and husband, sometimes in anger and sometimes in grief. Your contributions to this study of organ transplantation offer hope for people's future happiness. I really appreciate and admire your courage and I will never forget your narratives.

Thank you to all my mentors during my studies and research: Professor Masayoshi Tarui (Keio University), Professor Kyoko Tamura (Showa

University), Dr. Hiroshi Oda (Hokkaido University), Dr. Kimio Miyatake (Hokkaido University), and Professor Akihiro Sakai (Obirin University). Dr. Hiroyoshi Fujita and Dr. Takeshi Inoue also supported me constantly in the Hokkaido University Medical School during good days and bad!

Thank you to the mentors and staff of the Japanese and American academic institutions that stimulated my ideas and encouraged my tough back-and-forth inquiries between Japan and North America since 2000. My research began when I met Dr. Linda Hogle (University of Wisconsin) in San Francisco on my first visit to the United States and she has constantly encouraged me from across the ocean. Dr. Margaret Lock (McGill University) offered me great advice and some Japanese words to keep in mind that inspired me when I visited her office on my first trip to Canada. Dr. Marcia Inhorn (Yale University) has given me not only academic mentorship but also friendly encouragement whenever I feel I have hit a brick wall, and makes me want to come back to the United States at any time. The late Dr. Yukihiko Nose (Baylor College of Medicine) opened my eyes with his attitude to Japanese researchers in the United States, which had a strong impact on me, and his words of wisdom have remained with me. Dr. Katherine Ott (Smithsonian Institution) opened up many opportunities for me, along with Ms. Judy Chelnick: their friendly advice and the resources of world-leading research institutions such as the Smithsonian, Library of Congress, and NIH in the Washington, D.C., area stimulated my ideas and helped me to continue from my first small step in Japan through numerous challenges. Dr. Kirsten Shrader-Frechette (University of Notre Dame) encouraged me, not only as a bioethical specialist but also as a female researcher, with practical advice based on her own experiences as a female pioneer. I have also had great opportunities to work with people outside my field, such as in pharmaceutical companies: their points of view are very vivid and helpful, especially one of my business partners, Mr. Masaki Kanehira (a medical representative) and his colleagues, who motivated me and helped me to discover new horizons. I also received great support and my eyes were opened to a new field through my father's death and his funeral in Aoyagi Ceremonial Hall. Meeting and observing the layers-out, who are specialists in dealing with bereaved families, with their combination of the traditional and modern aspects of their work gave me great ideas for my own research. Their kindness encouraged me, especially President Shouji Yuasa and Mr. Akitoshi Sugihara, who contributed their expert knowledge via both interview and performance, offering valuable insight into traditional barriers to organ donation in Japan.

Thank you to the staff of Lexington Books: Ms. Alyc Helms found my presentation on "Rebirthable Life: Various Patterns of Japanese Brain-Dead Donors' Lives"—she emailed me and met with my American mentor, Dr. Terence Lyons, in 2008 and I started writing. Unfortunately cancer claimed my mentor in 2011 and I gave up on the book for a time, but luckily Ms. Amy King gave me another chance. Since English is not my first language, Ms. Lydia Wanstall copyedited the text; thanks to Amy and Lydia, I completed my first book.

Finally, to my special friend Yuko, who was fighting organ transplantation, rejection, and re-dialysis while I was in both Japan and North America: your friendship for me and your love for all humans gives me the energy for all of my work. Thank you always.

ONE

Introduction

It's good to know that organ donation has helped the recipients. It's all for the best if I don't know who received my son's organs and where; what's important is that everyone gets well. In fact, organ donation means "rebirthable life" for recipients. —A donor mother's narrative

Organ transplantation from brain-dead donors is an emerging medical technology that has created a number of social, legal, philosophical, ethical, and cultural issues throughout the world. It has often been pointed out that cultural issues in Japan are the main reason that barriers have been created, stalling the progress of brain-dead organ transplantation in the country (Abe 1994). A new organ transplantation law was legally approved in 1997; however, the cultural issues surrounding the medical practice remain unresolved, even following the law's revision in 2010. The first brain-dead transplant was performed in Japan in 1999, but to date (October 30, 2014), only 290 operations have been completed (for more information on the Japanese organ transplantation law, see appendix).

The number of concerned parties to organ transplantation has steadily increased over the years. This includes both people who have been involved in the process (recipients, living donors, and donor families) and medical staff engaged in transplantation by profession (surgeons, recipient coordinators, donor coordinators, and so on). Public differences of opinion and even arguments about brain-dead transplantation, however, appear a long way from reaching resolution, and the perceived problems and complications associated with it continue to increase. While mass media rush to cover organ transplantation stories at hospitals, the information they impart is often not only incorrect but also presented in soap opera fashion, succeeding only in distancing the general Japanese public

1

from the real-world events. Brain-dead organ transplantation has still failed to reach social consensus in Japan (see figure 1.1).

Organ transplantation is a form of advanced medical care, which can be divided into three categories:

1. Care for the birth of life, including reproductive medicine such as external fertilization—thanks to developments in this field, many infertile couples are able to have babies.
2. Care for quality of life, including organ transplantation—patients with organ failure can now live longer or their quality of life can be improved with a donated organ, but human donors are necessary for patients to receive this treatment.
3. Care for the end of life—this includes both life-sustaining medical treatment and the concept of respecting the dignity of a patient by hastening the end of their life: recently, making "living wills" has become more popular in Japan, which is also useful to ameliorate the quality of life of patients in hospices.

This book focuses on the topic of brain-dead organ transplantation, a cutting-edge medical treatment related to quality of life, and considers the type of medical care it offers. In addition, it considers the importance of grasping clues about how this emerging technology has transformed people's concept of life and death, which is strongly connected with tra-

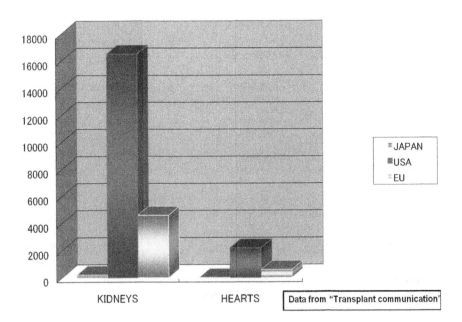

Figure 1.1.   Organ Donation 2008.

ditional beliefs, such as belief in life after death and similar. Because brain-dead organ transplantation is a relatively unknown medical treatment, there are few studies that focus on the issues surrounding it, such as transplant surgeons' dilemmas, recipients' guilt, and donor families' grief. The aim is of this book is to investigate these, which are very natural human feelings worldwide, but which may be affected by differences in culture, producing a variety of concepts of life and death in different parts of the globe.

Although many medical advances have been accepted over the years, the rapid development of medicine since the twentieth century has given rise to criticism, alarm, and concerns about runaway medical technology from professionals within the disciplines of medicine, law, bioethics, and religion, as well as the media. Little research has yet been done into the types of divisive problems created by emerging medical technologies such as brain-dead organ transplantation, how their acceptance has been gained, and what they have brought to Japanese society and culture. For example the traditional Japanese medical system, local beliefs and values, the Japanese concept of life and death, and especially the unique historical context of organ transplantation in Japan, including scandalous cases, have all molded the cultural acceptance or rejection of organ transplantation.

In our modern age it seems that refusal of advanced medical treatment is "just not realistic" (Awaya 2002: 110), although it should be noted that some see organ transplantation as an "enhancement" rather than a medical treatment. As a result, how has our concept of life fluctuated, how do we negotiate between this and the culture and traditions of our society, and how do we accept these fluctuations? To grasp the current situation it is necessary to research and gather narrative data from concerned parties and to analyze it carefully, using the qualitative research method. This will lead to a greater understanding of the transformation by advanced medical care of our concept of life in the past, present, and future.

I had two key questions when I was a student, one concerning brain death and the other concerning organ replacement. Brain death is a very ambiguous situation: is a human whose brain has died but whose heart is still beating dead or alive? Similarly, organ replacement creates an ambiguous human body: partly "self" and partly "other." Is the recipient one person or a hybrid cyborg combining two people? In 1997, when the first organ transplantation law was established in Japan, my patients were full of hope about brain-dead organ transplantation to enable them to survive but my colleagues—especially medical and law students—had a negative reaction. Why was this? The second Japanese organ transplant was performed in 1999 and I also felt a sense of discomfort at the news. I therefore started my research into brain-dead transplantation issues in 2000. Since this was three years after the new law, I expected that all my informants would be concerned parties to brain-dead organ donation, but just one year after the second heart transplant, there had only been twenty cases of brain-dead transplantation in Japan.

FIELDWORK

When I started my research into brain death and organ transplantation, I learned how naïve the questions and design of my research were. I simply thought that I should learn what brain death and organ transplantation mean to the concerned parties, such as transplant surgeons, organ recipients, and donor families, but immediately hit a stumbling block. How was I to contact the concerned parties? There is no interrelationship between anthropology departments (faculty of letters) and medical schools to facilitate contact with transplant surgeons. How was I to get to know organ recipients? Hospitals keep personal information strictly confidential to protect their patients' privacy. How could I contact the donor families? Even recipients are not permitted to write a thank you letter directly, in order to respect the anonymity of organ donation. This was the first barrier in my research.

I started volunteering in an organ transplant organization, where I met various recipients who had received organs from living donors, heart-dead donors after ten years of waiting, and overseas (brain-dead) transplants. Each had various unexpected and complex experiences to recount. This organization holds a special event called the "Transplant Games," to which it invites donor families as guests to show recipients' gratitude for the donated organs. Another aim of the organization is to build mutual understanding between recipients and donor families in a public place with medical staff through the Japan Organ Transplant Network (JOTN). Through volunteering work, I also had the opportunity to get to know some donor families, who told me of their own unpredictable and extraordinary experiences. Unfortunately, the relationship between the recipients and donor families exhibited serious tensions. In addition, I met transplant surgeons, who were working as mediators between donor families and recipients. I decided that although I could not describe the ethnography of the world of concerned parties to brain-dead transplantation, I should describe the changing world they experienced after 2000 as the new law began to take effect. Although everyone I encountered was very friendly and kind individually, they had strong biased views about each other and this invited misunderstandings. I hope that the work of anthropologists, especially narrative research, may help to support their mutual understanding in the future.

I have been investigating the effects of brain-dead transplantation on human beings now for more than ten years, collating my initial research and findings in my PhD thesis (Yasuoka 2006), and continuing follow-up research since then.[1]

In this book, I describe the restarted brain-dead transplantation world in Japan from 2000 to 2014. I have conducted interview research among concerned parties to organ transplantation, including transplant surgeons, recipients, and donor families. I have listened carefully to gather narrative data and tried to investigate further to bring their responses to this advanced medical treatment into sharp relief. How do they describe their experiences of brain-dead organ transplantation, and what difference has it made to their daily lives and outlooks? The analysis and discussion of their narratives is divided into the following three sections:

1. Transplant surgeons' ambivalence toward brain-dead organ transplantation
2. Recipients' experiences of organ reception
3. Donor families' decisions surrounding organ donation

It is clear from the narratives that the new concept of "brain death" required for living organ transplantation has changed concerned parties' concepts of life and death. I explore the differences in perception and the friction caused by such new concepts of life for concerned parties from both within and outside the transplantation "community." My research particularly focuses on the difficulties encountered by recipients and donor families as they approach the issue of organ transplantation from opposite sides (as receivers and givers) and how these can create tensions between them as they reconstruct their "concepts of life" after the process. By analyzing and discussing these findings, I hope this research will become the cornerstone of further study into the transformation and future direction of people's concepts of life.

HISTORY OF ORGAN TRANSPLANTATION IN JAPAN

The replacement of human body parts has a long history, dating back to antiquity. Supplying lost or failed parts of a human body with new materials (such as artificial legs or teeth) or replacing them with human tissue (such as skin and corneas) is now common practice. These, however, are not the inner organs of the body, so they don't need either treatment with drugs to suppress the immune system to decrease the risk of rejection or organ donation from brain-dead donors. Since humans will die without the function of their key organs—heart, liver, kidneys, and so on—great efforts have long continued in medical science to discover suitable replacements.

Artificial organs were invented in the nineteenth century, and soon gained popularity, but they were not replacements for the major organs yet due to the barrier of promoting blood clots and causing stroke or other serious diseases. The most successful artificial organ in current use is kidney dialysis, which has been saving patients' lives since around 1945, working via a machine outside the body. The liver, however, is a very complex organ and there is no prospect currently of an artificial liver emerging on the market. A self-contained total artificial heart already exists, but the biggest barrier to its use for patients is that they may be "clot-prone," in which case the recipient will die: the artificial heart is not yet as successful as human heart transplantation (Project Bionics 2014).

Organ transplantation is a medical treatment that saves lives by replacing a patient's failed organ with a healthy human (or animal) one (Medical Information Network Society 2014). Medical science advanced a great deal in the twentieth century, including in the field of organ transplantation, but it simultaneously produced many unexpected and difficult issues, and these are especially prevalent in Japan. Japan has the severest organ shortage in the world (as a result of the lowest organ donation number) and there is still no social consensus about the meaning of brain death. These ongoing problems stem from the unique history of Japanese organ transplantation compared to other countries, and it is suspected as a cause of delaying organ transplant medical treatment throughout the world.

The first Japanese heart transplant was performed by Dr. Juro Wada in 1968, just a year after the world's first heart transplant had been conducted by Dr. Christian Barnard in Cape Town in South Africa (Japan Organ Transplant Network 2014). This was a very early success story of heart transplantation compared with other countries, but the second Japanese heart transplant did not take place until 1999, after a total intermission of thirty-one years. During this time, various huge developments and changes took place in the organ transplantation medical arena on a global scale outside Japan, with rapid and vast expansions (see table 1.1). Japanese organ transplant treatment, however, developed in a unique way, relying only on living donors and cadaveric and overseas transplants.

Japanese organ transplant research began in the early twentieth century with a paper titled "Organ Transplantation," presented in Kyoto by Hansaku Yamauchi, a pioneer of research through experimentation with cats and dogs. The first kidney transplant in Japan was in 1956 (two years after the world's first kidney transplant): a diseased kidney was transplanted, using an anuric patient's thigh artery and vein, as a temporary emergency treatment until the patient was able to self-produce urine again and the organ was removed (see table 1.2). The first Japanese liver transplant was conducted in 1964 (the year following the world's first liver transplant), but the recipient died after only five days. The second

Table 1.1.

1954	The first kidney transplant by Joseph E. Murray and John Merrill in Boston, USA
1963	The first liver transplant by Thomas Starzl in Denver, USA
1967	The first heart transplant by Christian Barnard in Cape Town, South Africa
1968	The first Japanese heart transplant by Juro Wada in Sapporo
1969	Denton Cooley, in the first clinical application of the total artificial heart, implants a pneumatically powered heart designed by Domingo Liotta (from the laboratory of Michael DeBakey) in Houston, USA as a bridge to transplantation into a forty-seven-year-old male, who survives sixty-four hours on the total artificial heart and thirty-two hours following transplantation
1988	The first partial liver transplant from a living donor by Silvano Raia in São Paulo, Brazil
1989	The first Japanese partial liver transplant from a living donor by Naofumi Nagasue in Shimane

such operation was performed in 1969, but then cadaveric liver transplantation was interrupted until 1993.

The first heart transplant operation took place in 1968 (the year following the world's first heart transplant), but this great achievement in Japanese medical history turned into a murder investigation, known as the "Wada case" (see table 1.3).

Several accusations were made in this case. The organ donor, a victim of drowning, was still alive and might have recovered if given sufficient medical attention—he recovered spontaneous breathing in the ambulance but Dr. Wada administered a muscle relaxant to harvest the heart on the patient's arrival at the hospital. In addition, the recipient's heart condition was not sufficiently critical to require a heart transplant. Finally, the fact that Dr. Wada carried out both the brain death evaluation of the donor and the selection of the recipient was yet another cause for concern.

In 2010, the late Dr. Y. Nose, a Japanese artificial organ inventor working in Houston, Texas, and involved in Project Bionics (Project Bionics 2014), gave further details about the case. He said that he had spoken with Dr. Wada on the phone from the United States at the time and had advised against the operation. Dr. Wada had not listened but had gone ahead with the operation because he wanted to do the first heart transplant in Japan, and not because of medical need. Dr. Wada is known as "the blackest white" (black for guilt, and white for innocence: he is legally innocent due to lack of evidence, because he destroyed all documents pertaining to the case, but Japanese public opinion believes in his guilt). Unfortunately, both Dr. Wada and Dr. Nose have passed away and the truth of the "Wada case" was lost with them.

Table 1.2.

1956	The first kidney transplant by Takamitsu Kusumoto in Niigata
1964	The first liver transplant by Seiji Kimoto in Tokyo
1968	The first heart transplant by Juro Wada in Sapporo
1997	Organ transplantation law established
1999	First organ donation from brain-dead donor under the new law
2010	January 17—"family-first organ donor rule" implemented*
2010	July 17—revision of organ transplantation law implemented

* On the latest revised Japanese donor card, if the holder wishes to use the "family-first organ donor rule," he or she should write the name of the recipient in the special comment column (Japan Organ Transplant Network, 2014).

I have lived in Sapporo since 1975 and visit Ishikari beach every summer, as do many of my students, my friends, and family members: summer is very short in Sapporo and people enjoy the beach after the long winter. Most of them know very little about the details of the "Wada case," but in fact the first Japanese brain-dead donor drowned on Ishikari beach, and the heart recipient received the organ in Sapporo Medical School Hospital in 1968.

After these events, Japanese organ transplantation (heart and liver) stopped for thirty-one years, as a result of feelings of resistance and worry toward brain-dead transplantation, compared to attitudes in the West (Japan Organ Transplant Network 2014). Most heart and liver transplants therefore relied on overseas surgery, and most kidney transplants relied on living donors inside the family circle in Japan or in developing south Asian countries where organ tourism is becoming an increasing problem. Various ethical issues arise from both overseas and living donor transplantation, which can lead to human right issues on an international scale as well as familial, domestic, and societal problems within Japan. The World Health Organization (WHO) raised concern about "organ tracking" problems, and in the Istanbul Declaration of 2008 called for "organ self-sufficiency." As a result, many countries including Australia prohibited overseas transplants and Japanese recipients had fewer opportunities to receive organs abroad.

A British medical anthropologist working in Canada, Dr. Lock, pointed out that the low levels of organ donation and the passive attitude toward brain death in Japan are a direct fallout from the "Wada case," which caused huge side-effects for Japanese people, including a great deal of mistrust (Lock 2002). My research data, expanding on Dr. Lock's findings, show that two kinds of mistrust are prevalent in Japan: the first is a mistrust of brain-dead organ transplant medical care itself, and the second is a mistrust of doctors, and especially transplant surgeons like

Table 1.3.

1968	August—heart transplant by Juro Wada in Sapporo December—Dr. Wada faced criminal prosecution by various medical specialists—the recipient died after eighty-three days because he wasn't a suitable heart transplant candidate
1970	Dr. Wada charged with the crimes of murder, professional negligence, and illegally disposing of a body, but all cases later dropped because of insufficient evidence, leading to an "innocent" verdict
1973	Dr. Wada warned by Japan Federation of Bar Associations (JFBA) about the validity of the heart transplant operation
1997	Original organ transplantation law established in Japan
1999	First brain-dead transplant performed under the new law in Japan (the second heart transplant after the "Wada case," after thirty-one years' intermission)
2011	Dr. Wada dies—the truth of the "Wada case" will never now be uncovered

Dr. Wada (Yasuoka 2013). The former is of crucial significance because organ transplant treatment relies on organ donations with the consent of donors and/or donor families in a spirit of love and goodwill.

THE CURRENT SITUATION REGARDING BRAIN DEATH AND ORGAN TRANSPLANTATION IN JAPAN

The "Wada case" still resonates today and is one reason for the Japanese problem of infrequent organ donation, among other unique social and cultural issues. Although there are strong doubts about whether the case was in fact a suitable brain-dead organ transplant, it offered a ray of hope for many end-stage organ failure patients who felt they were under sentence of death. Nevertheless, some patients still felt that they would rather die with dignity than accept this new treatment of someone else's body part, which they felt would bring disgrace on them. People all over Japan paid attention to the details and the case attracted tremendous interest at the time. When Dr. Wada was charged with capital murder, even though the prosecution eventually dropped the charge, the history of Japanese organ transplantation suffered a hiatus for thirty-one years as a result.

In the 1980s the immunosuppressant cyclosporine was developed, and a boom in organ transplantation took place in the United States, reinstituting brain-dead organ transplantation after a period during which the majority of recipients had suffered organ rejection, making the treatment unpopular. The Japanese Society for Transplantation launched an advertising campaign for brain-dead transplantation in 1982, having argued for fifteen years about whether brain-dead status constituted human death. Because of this, "The Brain Death Ad Hoc Commission on Administrative Reform" was set up in March 1990. Nevertheless, many

Japanese people still feel uncertain about recognizing brain death as human death because of traditional cultural issues surrounding the warm body, still-beating heart, and retention of color in the face of the brain-dead person.

Japan's first organ transplantation law came into effect in October 1997, stating that only in the case of someone donating organs for transplantation is brain death to be considered human death. From that day, brain-dead organ transplantation was reinstituted to fill in the "missing piece" of advanced medical treatment, and the first brain-dead organ transplant took place in 1999. Only eighty-six transplants from brain-dead donors took place under the original Japanese organ transplantation law (October 16, 1997–July 16, 2010), however, and only 204 brain-dead transplants have been performed even since the law was revised in July 2010—a total of 290 cases up to October 30, 2014. According to a medical anthropologist in North America, organ donation numbers from brain-dead donors are still at a very low level in Japan because of the fallout from the "Wada case" (Lock 2002).

Organ shortages are not only a Japanese problem but a worldwide one, yet the organ donation rates in Japan are by far the lowest among medically advanced countries. Another unusual phenomenon has also arisen recently: although the number of Japanese people holding donor cards or donation wills has gone up, the number of actual organ donations has decreased. One frequently mentioned cultural issue concerns the fact that Japanese people have a high level of respect for the integrity of the dead body, but it is hard to consider that this concept alone is the cause of the low rate of organ donations. This phenomenon shows that while Japan has advanced medical technology, Japanese people do not find it so easy to adapt to modern practices, retaining old-fashioned traditional beliefs about the dead body and death itself.

The Japanese organ shortage is not only deadly to patients awaiting treatment; it has also created a knock-on effect internationally, with issues such as overseas transplantation, which includes worldwide medical tourism problems. Under Japan's original organ transplantation law, organ donations from children under fifteen years old were banned, and child patients had to rely on living donors or overseas transplantation (under the current revised law all ages can donate). This meant that the only way for a Japanese child to receive a heart transplant was via overseas surgery, and many patients lost their lives while waiting for an organ in foreign countries, returning to Japan only after death (Arimura 1999).

Even the existence of medical staff dedicated to organ transplantation and the details of their roles are generally unknown in Japan because the medical world is veiled from ordinary people as a tight-knit group of doctors in a closed corporate culture society. Japanese organ transplant staff has their hands full with not only their jobs but also various voluntary activities: they are frequently involved in campaigns to enlighten and edify the public about organ donation and transplantation issues, often without pay and giving up their free time to do so. Because of the Wada case, Japanese people have mistrusted organ transplantation, especially transplant surgeons, so few know about the surgeons' modest but faithful volunteer activities. According to a medical representative's narrative, "There are many problems surrounding organ transplantation in Japan but the worst thing is *indifference* to the issue."

Before the new organ transplantation law was established in 1997, surgeons would ensure that harvested organs would stay within the same hospital, but afterwards the Japan Organ Transplant Network took control of donated organs to maintain "fairness." Thus, a donor's organ from a hospital in Tokyo (central Japan) might be given to a recipient in Okinawa (southern Japan) or Sapporo (northern Japan), and the Tokyo hospital has no priority for receiving any organ donated within its theatres under revised law. (Before the 1997 law, there was an unwritten rule in hospitals concerning kidney donations, which stated, "Keep one, ship one," meaning that one kidney was retained for the donor's hospital and the other was sent to another hospital.) As a result, surgeons' motivation for organ harvesting lessened because they did not know whether the organ would be given to a patient in their own hospital; this is considered a contributory factor in the low rate of organ donation in Japan.

The new law's agenda placed great weight on such operations being equitable and externally justified, as well as on transparency. The role of transplantation coordinator was introduced to ensure that the law's strictures were strictly observed. There are two kinds: donor coordinators and recipient coordinators. Recipient coordinators are licensed clinical nurses—they coordinate transplantation from the perspective of recipients and take care of recipients before and after the operation. Donor coordinators do not need a clinical nurse license—if they administer an injection to a donor it is only after death, so this is not necessary. However, they have to coordinate the process smoothly from confirming brain death to completing organ transplantation in the recipient, including coordinating with donor families, which is an extremely difficult aspect of the role.

These new roles give us further clues from the perspective of medical staff about Japanese people's responses to the new practice of organ transplantation. My mission in this book, after all, is not to uncover the details of the traumatic history of organ transplantation in Japan: my research examines patients and their reactions to and feelings about the medical issues surrounding organ transplantation. A medical anthropologist's task is to trace transplant surgeons and coordinators, organ recipients and donor families, listen to their narratives, write their ethnography, and analyze the data gathered to uncover information about the situation in which they find themselves. Such information helps other patients and bereaved families who feel that they are in a hopeless situation. I have also had the opportunity to follow up my research with twenty-three concerned parties from my first interviews in 2002 to date, to better grasp how their stories are developing over the years. These additional data may focus the direction of organ transplantation research in the future, shedding some light onto how to deal with the treatment and the relationships between concerned parties as the medical technology continues to develop.

REACTIONS TO ORGAN TRANSPLANTATION IN JAPAN

In this book I consider how human beings might construct better relationships with emerging medical technology in the twenty-first century in the light of the twentieth century's medical advances. I introduce the narratives of Japanese concerned parties to organ transplantation (transplant medical staff including transplant surgeons, recipient coordinators and a donor coordinator, recipients, and donor families) and present ethnography of both emerging medical technology and reactions to the processes of organ donation and reception through these data. By paying attention to the various viewpoints of the three categories of concerned party, perspective research into brain-dead organ transplantation becomes possible.

Japan is one of the world's most medically developed countries and has saved many internal patients' lives, as well as assisting patients from developing countries, but organ transplantation is still an enormous issue. The whole world is facing a severe organ shortage, and Japan's situation is the worst in this regard. In fact, since the transplantation law was revised, the total number of organ donations has been increasing more slowly than had been envisaged and kidney donations from brain-dead donors have even been decreasing. Despite advanced medical technology and highly skilled transplant surgeons, many organ recipient candidates are on a long waiting list and too few organ donations are offered from brain-dead donors (via donation wills or donor family consent) to meet the demand.

In general, Japanese people admire cutting-edge medical technology and expect to defeat pernicious diseases, approving of the development of advanced medical technology and the hope it offers patients diagnosed with a fatal disease. In Sapporo in particular (in northern Japan, an area that is less traditional and conservative, and freer from constraints than southwestern Japan) people are very rational and adapt quickly to new ideas with an easy openness. Initially, the new technology of organ transplantation from brain-dead donors appeared to provide surgeons with an opportunity to make the impossible possible and save their fatally ill patients. In 1968, at the time of the first heart transplant in Japan, my mother made mental notes on the sensational news on the radio, but it was entirely welcome. The treatment was seen as effective and very attractive; there was even a tendency to deify transplant surgeons (Setoyama 2001). The first transplant surgeons who came back to Japan having worked in the United States were seen as having "the hands of God" and were treated like movie stars, but the low numbers of transplants meant that attention waned both in the medical world and among the public as reports about them became sparser (Todo 2000).

During the long intermission in its organ transplant medical service, however, Japan progressed in a completely different and twisted way from other medically developed countries. The "Wada case" was highly sensational at the time and was all over the news, causing a heightened sensitivity to the issue and inviting drama. Simultaneously, however, it was perceived as science fiction rather than real-life medical progress, and the public seemed almost to take organ transplant issues for granted, showing interest only in the sensational aspects but not understanding the details. Such attitudes toward both organ transplantation issues and the topic of brain death remain current because death is a taboo subject in Japanese society.

In 1999, at the time of the first transplant under the new Japanese organ transplantation law (which was only the second heart transplant in Japan), I was a student preparing to start organ transplant research in graduate school, so I remember the day vividly. I will never forget that blue cold box used to deliver organs from a donor to plural recipients across Japan by coordinators who were airlifted to hospital by helicopter. Everybody was glued to the television, hardly believing what they were seeing. This was the first organ delivery from a brain-dead donor under the new law, despite the fact that it had been on the statute book for two years. Having thought that the main barrier to organ donation was a legal one, it became apparent after the new law was instituted that the main issues were social and cultural ones (combined with the stringent requirements of the 1997 law).

According to my mother's reminiscences and my experience, the reactions of the Japanese people to these events of 1968 and 1999 were not very different. During the intervening thirty-one years there had been no heart transplant cases, but Japan had changed from a developing to a developed country after World War II and was thus used to rapid progress and modernization in daily life. Both events were very sensational, attracting conspicuous attention from the media, which, however, gave inadequate information and treated the stories more as soap opera–style news than medical progress. It seems that organ transplantation from brain-dead donors is not only a medical matter but also a cultural issue. By focusing on the cultural aspects of the problem, therefore, I believe that we may find new data to help solve the issue in a positive way.

Even despite the interest in and hopes for brain-dead organ transplantation, somehow it appears to leave a nasty taste in people's mouths. It is, after all, a mysterious medical treatment in which life and death intersect, and it cannot take place without the outside agent of the donor. It is difficult to reconcile the idea of the wonderful high-technology treatment of the "gift of life" with the fact that the process relies on a person's death, transferring to the organ recipient the guilt of being associated not only with that death but also with the grief of the donor's family. And can it really be a "gift of life" if some Japanese recipients have to beg on street corners to raise the money to receive such treatment abroad that they cannot get at home? In addition, organ transplantation involves many people, compared with reproductive medicine and dignified death: the former is a very private marital issue and the latter is reflected and rooted in personal values. In organ transplantation, the donor's organ is donated to another person, the recipient is gifted another person's organ and the transplant surgeon transplants one person's organ into another. It is fundamentally different from other branches of medicine and we need to try to incorporate it into conventional medicine carefully because of its different perspective. I hope that in the future the combination of cutting-edge and conventional medicine may make such processes smoother and easier for all involved, with no conflicts between the proponents of either, causing difficulties for their patients.

The original Japanese organ transplantation law, established in 1997, was unique in a positive and a negative way, and caused Japan to have the lowest organ donation numbers in the world. It was introduced after the long intermission (1969–1996) in organ transplantation in the country, and in fact it is considered the strictest transplantation law in the world—this strictness is one reason why the organ donation numbers are so low. Although the "Wada case" left the side effect that many Japanese people mistrust both organ transplantation itself and medical doctors (Lock 2002), it also gave the country time to think over brain death and organ transplantation issues (Fox and Swazey 1992). In spite of this background and the unique history of organ transplantation in Japan, most Japanese people do not try to discuss such fundamental human issues of life and death.

Within the law:

1. Brain death was considered human death only when the patient had agreed to donate organs in the case of brain-dead status.
2. Donation wills were required of both the patient and his/her family.
3. Donations by children under fifteen years of age were prohibited.

Thus, brain-dead status was considered human death only if the patient had an organ donation will; for non-organ donors, only heart death was considered the end of human life. This invited the criticism that both the law and the Japanese definition of brain death were ambiguous, and since the definition is only in use in the case of organ harvesting (not in day-to-day life) it can be seen as a very utilitarian theory (Nakajima 2000).

So these definitions are for organ harvest not for Japanese humans, so it is rational and utilitarian focus is only on organ harvest.

There is still no formal definition of brain death in Japan, even under the new law (prior to which there was an unspoken understanding that human death was heart death). The new criterion of brain death arose from the emerging technology of organ donation; prior to the procedure's availability no status of "brain-dead" was required. The fact that this change is relatively recent and associated with such cutting-edge and therefore relatively unknown technology is likely to contribute to the population's opposing views and concerns about brain death.

Innovative medical technology has mostly been welcomed by people (particularly users such as patients) in Japan, but in some cases matters of preference strongly connected with Japanese society, culture, traditions, and ethics have moved people to turn against such advances. The accelerating speed at which important medical advances have arrived since the latter part of the twentieth century has produced unpredictable shifts and situations. The more medical technology innovates, the more we should focus on the "explanatory model" (Kleinman 1980 and 1988). This is one method used by medical anthropologists to shed light on emerging medical technology via concerned parties' narratives, retaining objectivity and understanding individuals' clinical experiences, then analyzing the findings through qualitative research.

Using the "explanatory model," cutting-edge technology to negotiate traditional and cultural models in our daily life could be incorporated into conventional medicine by creating a deeper understanding. We cannot help but feel some confusion when we try to change our concepts of life and death as a result of new medical issues such as brain death or organ transplantation, but we should try to overcome the discord between conservative opinions and groundbreaking views, and move from confrontation to cooperation. Nevertheless, we cannot accept a new definition of human death or innovative medical care blindly; that would be unrealistic. We have to grasp a better way, through struggle, trial, and error, to manage the conflict effectively and try to find a method of incorporating the innovations into ordinary life.

We need to focus attention on the "explanatory model" of medical brain-dead transplant care and reveal the narratives of concerned parties to organ transplantation in Japan. This will illuminate their interpretations and ideas, and thus highlight the surrounding cultural and ethical phenomena and the grave problems arising, and reveal the mystery of humans. My initial interview research revealed that the narratives of concerned parties were too sensational, too complex, and too unique for non-concerned parties to understand their individual concepts of life and death with their own rationalization. It also indicated that we need to try to understand not only human concepts of life and death but also Japanese culture, tradition, and religious beliefs, and how they have mixed with various opposing elements from the West in Japan since the country's defeat in World War II.

1. For transplant surgeons: how does a medical profession that has a key role in organ transplantation embrace the ambivalence of the procedure—both giving and taking life?
2. For recipients: how do they give both social and cultural meaning to their experience of organ transplantation and how do they accept their own experience of living with a transplanted organ?
3. For donor families: can we use the "explanatory model" to understand their conflicting feelings and unique responses to their situation as they grieve their loved ones while offering the "gift of life" to others?

It is necessary to understand the hidden messages within their narratives and interpret their words both logically and emotionally while bearing in mind their social and cultural contexts. My interview research has investigated how these concerned parties have tried to reach acceptance and cope with the problems caused by such new medical technology in a practical manner. At the same time, it has shed light on the discrepancies in their concepts of life as a result of their involvement in organ transplantation, stemming from differences in their roles and involvement. This fruitful area of research may help others to construct better relationships with emerging medical technology and thereby reduce some of the burning issues surrounding organ transplantation in Japan.

NOTE

1. During the writing of this book (2008–2014), I had a great opportunity to learn further personal narrative data from concerned parties and I also use this in the text.

REFERENCES

Abe, T. (1994). "Cultural Theory of Life." In *Why Is Brain-Dead Transplantation a Problem? Messages from Medical Doctors against the Brain-Dead Transplantation Law*, edited by Y. Watanabe and T. Abe, 219–221. Tokyo: Yumiru Publisher.
Arimura, H. (1999). *Not Received a Gift*. Tokyo: Keizaikai Co. Ltd.
Awaya, T. (2002). "Exploitation of Resources and Commercialization of Human Body and Modern Human Body Ownership." *Associé* 9: 101–112.
Fox, R., and Swazey, J. (1992). *Spare Parts: Organ Replacement in American Society*. New York: Oxford University Press.
Japan Organ Transplant Network. (2014). "The History of Transplanting" [website]. http://www.jotnw.or.jp/english/01.html, accessed 09/30/2014.

Kleinman, A. (1980). *Patients and Healers in the Context of Culture: An Exploration of the Borderland between Anthropology, Medicine, and Psychiatry*. Oakland: University of California Press.

———. (1988). *The Illness Narratives: Suffering, Healing and the Human Condition*. New York: Basic Books.

Kyodo News Service: Organ Transplant Group of Reporters of City News. (1998). *A Frozen Heart*. Tokyo: Kyodo News Service.

Lock, M. (2002). *Twice Dead: Organ Transplants and the Reinvention of Death*. Berkeley: University of California Press.

Medical Information Network Society. (2014). "Transplant Communication" [website]. http://www.medi-net.or.jp/tcnet/index_e.html, accessed 04/17/2014.

Nakajima, M. (2000). *Brain Death and Organ Transplantation Law* [paperback pocket edition]. Tokyo: Bungeishunju Ltd.

Project Bionics, Artificial Organs from Discovery to Clinical Use: An ASAIO History Project at The Smithsonian [website]. http://echo.gmu.edu/bionics, accessed 04/17/2014.

Setoyama, M. (2001). "My Recommended 10 Best Books for Students and Residents." *Medical Community Weekly World Newspaper* 16(4): 24–34.

Todo, S. (2000). "Key People of the 21st Century." *Yomiuri Year Book 2000*. Tokyo: The Yomiuri Shimbun.

Yasuoka, M. K. (2006). "Rebirthable Life: Medical Anthropology Study of the Concept of Life According to Concerned Parties Involved in Brain Death and Organ Transplantation." PhD thesis: Department of History and Anthropology (Medical Anthropology), Graduate School of Letters, Hokkaido University, Sapporo, Japan (unpublished).

———. (2011). "Revision of Organ Transplantation Law in Japan: Brain Death, Presumed Consent, and Donation of Children's Organs." In *Applied Ethics: Old Wine in New Bottles?* Center for Applied Ethics and Philosophy, 186–198. Sapporo, Japan: Center for Applied Ethics and Philosophy, Hokkaido University.

———. (2013). "Rebirthable Life: Narratives and Reproductive Life of Japanese Brain-Dead Donors." *Research Journal of Graduate Students of Letters* 8: 73–81.

TWO

Narratives of Transplant Surgeons and Coordinators

INTRODUCTION

Why organ transplant? I want to save people. Because I want to save patients who are abandoned by others. It is a story that I work as all the treatment except organ transplant. I don't want to do organ transplant. The patients are happiest if they do not undergo organ transplant and recover. If there isn't anything more to it than that I only say to do organ transplant. Well, it must be so. Because there is not it with such an easy thing. It is the very last treatment, because the complications should be developed, the medicines are also needed, that is, transplant medical care is not medical care to cure a disease of recipients and it is medical care to make recipients new disease. Though recipients were taken their heart and the heart changes of donor's and got well, organ transplant is medical care to make organ recipients new disease to take an immunosuppressive drug and then they have risk to suffer from infectious disease. Such a medical care has unreasonableness. There is unreasonableness even if I intend not to be able to happen as much as possible. If I do not do organ transplant to patients and they recovered, I try to choose at first to make the medical care that is not, and I try to save the other patients who is not helped other medical treatment somehow. Consequential medical treatment. Treatment of the very last resort. —A transplant surgeon's narrative

The emerging medical technologies of the twentieth and twenty-first centuries have produced not only new medical treatments but also new experts, including organ transplant surgeons, recipient coordinators, and donor coordinators. This chapter examines the responses of these medical professionals to organ transplants from brain-dead donors and their thoughts about the innovative procedures they perform. It also investigates what drives them to work in the field of organ transplantation. The sections below set out the experts' reactions to organ transplantation treatment in Japan through the narratives, collected via formal interviews, of seven transplant surgeons and three coordinators (two recipients coordinators and one donor coordinator) who work with them.

All the surgeons and coordinators are proud of engaging professionally in organ transplantation. The transplant surgeons admire the field as a development of medical treatment and as a scientific innovation, although their individual feelings about organ transplantation vary somewhat depending on the organs they specialize in transplanting—whether heart, liver, or kidney. In a similar way, the narratives display the very different attitudes of recipient coordinators and donor coordinators. While recipient coordinators work with patients in a situation that offers expectation and hope, donor coordinators have to work with and support grieving donor families. Organ transplantation is not a simple treatment, but the professionals reveal the typical underlying responses of human love and hatred.

Although transplant surgeons and other medical staff actively decide on their profession as a result of various motivations, and undergo extensive education and training to achieve their ambition, they nevertheless face strong dilemmas working in the field. Recipients, donors, and donor families do not choose organ reception and donation; it is a choice imposed on them, and may well not be their preferred option. The emotional narratives of transplant surgeons and coordinators are very rarely obtained, but are extremely useful as they offer insight to enable a deeper understanding and a professional perspective on organ transplantation and its impacts on medicine more broadly. Unlike the patients involved and their families, the medical professionals have chosen to be concerned parties to organ transplantation.

Medical staff in Japan has to adjust to three particularly noteworthy changes as a result of organ transplantation.

1. This emerging medical technology has produced new jobs in unusual circumstances, and medical personnel have struggled to handle unexpected changes resulting from the transplantation of organs from a brain-dead donor to a recipient. A strong paternalistic relationship still exists between Japanese doctors and patients, but patients now have less automatic trust and faith in medical staff.

2. In Japanese medical environments, the power balance between doctors and other medical workers such as nurses have traditionally been uneven, but the role of each associated health professional is of vital importance in the field of organ transplantation. As a result, Japanese conventional medicine and the medical systems in Japanese hospitals have to change, since organ transplantation relies on medical care from a team of equals.

3. Organ transplantation forces a fundamental change on the doctor–patient relationship in Japan. This medical treatment requires a

radical reassessment of the structure of the traditional Japanese paternalistic medical relationship because medical doctors cannot help their patients (the recipients) without organs donated by donors with the acceptance of donor families (Yasuoka 2006).

AMBIVALENCE TOWARD ORGAN TRANSPLANTATION

Organ transplantation from brain-dead donors is a medical treatment that gives rise to very ambivalent reactions among concerned parties— even medical doctors. Japanese surgeons used to have a duty of care predominantly to their own patients; now they also have to think simultaneously about both the donor and the donor family. They value the "gift of life" organ transplantation offers recipients and feel it is part of the doctor's mission to save a patient. Unfortunately, though, the treatment relies on a harvested organ to save the recipient. When surgeons harvest a heart, removing it from a brain-dead but still living donor and holding it in their hands, they inevitably feel the sorrow and guilt associated with ending a life, even while they are trying to save another life.

The transplant surgeons' narratives reveal how much they have had to work on dealing with their guilt on behalf of the recipients and to make it their mission to transform understanding of the organ transplantation process, shedding new light on their position as surgeons. The paternalistic power of doctors in Japan was and often still is too strong for patients to talk with them as equals: most patients give up on the idea of informed consent and simply obey their doctor's advice, abandoning any pretense of autonomy. Organ transplantation is just one of many emerging medical technologies that have been turning the traditional way of seeing the medical world on its head: the donor is a new agent in this world, and is a formidable but unpredictable influence in both positive and negative ways.

Organ transplantation has had an extraordinary and unimaginable impact in the twenty-first century. Since ancient times, as a global society we have put great faith in wonderful advances in medicine and expected continual medical progress, hoping to overcome various deadly diseases and even death itself. Now, however, the issues arising from organ transplantation from brain-dead donors have slowed the hypergrowth of medical technologies. It is time to take a step back and rethink our attitudes to medicine and indeed to life and death. The transplant surgeons' narratives show that they have changed their role as paternalistic doctors, becoming the mediators between donors and recipients. Their responses give us an opportunity to examine seriously and try to understand both the impacts of new medical procedures and better ways to share our lives with emerging medical technologies.

REVIVING MEDICAL CARE: TRANSPLANTING ORGANS

In essence, transplant surgeons see organ transplantation from brain-dead donors as an admirable "gift of life" produced by emerging medical technology in the twentieth century and developing in the twenty-first century, offering great possibilities to make life better for human beings in the future. However the meaning of "gift of life" and the assessment of organ transplantation vary among surgeons, often relating to the organ in which they specialize. Most transplant surgeons were born and educated in Japan but they received specialized education about organ transplantation and gained experience saving recipients in the United States while training and working as organ transplantation specialists. They may thus have gained a more scientific mindset through their training but the Japanese culture and traditional beliefs are still deeply embedded.

1. Heart Transplant Surgeons

To harvest a beating heart and transplant it into a recipient, heart transplant surgeons have to rely on the availability of a brain-dead donor whose organs are still functioning. By law in Japan one surgeon should harvest the heart and another perform the transplant operation, but the number of specialist heart transplant surgeons is limited so one surgeon may have to perform both operations. Although heart transplant surgeons feel guilty when they harvest a beating heart from a brain-dead donor, they see organ transplantation as a wonderful procedure, giving hope to patients who would otherwise die. "Although we can save one heart recipient, I feel sad to lose a brain-dead donor whose beating heart I have to harvest: I feel that I gave them the finishing blow!" a transplant surgeon told me.

2. Liver Transplant Surgeons

Liver transplants are also mostly dependent on brain-dead donors; many Japanese recipients have to resort to an overseas transplant, usually in Australia. Live organ transplantation is possible; however, from a living donor inside the family circle, so many Japanese recipients' family members want to donate their organs. The risks from live liver organ transplants are much higher than from kidney transplants, not only for the recipient but also for the donor, but a donor without a heartbeat cannot donate a liver, making the procedure a difficult one. Most surgeons prefer to use brain-dead donors where possible because of the potential aggressive invasiveness of harvesting a liver from a living donor. Although liver transplant surgeons see the organ transplantation procedure as very stressful, their narratives show that they feel especially aware of the benefits of transplant medicine.

3. Kidney Transplant Surgeons

Kidney transplants are different from those of other organs such as heart, liver, and pancreas, and are currently recognized practically as standard medical care in Japan. Nevertheless, all kidney recipients have faced death and kidney transplant surgeons have a similar role to play to other transplant surgeons. For kidney transplant procedures options include transplantation from brain-dead donors, cadaveric donors, or living donors. Potential donation numbers are high because the human body has two kidneys so a dead donor can save two recipients and a living kidney donor has a better chance of survival than a living donor of a liver. Recipients are able to receive an organ on more than one occasion and patients are also able to live on dialysis (artificial kidneys).

4. Recipient Coordinators

Recipient coordinators or hospital coordinators organize organ transplants for recipients; they support them and their families during the transplantation process to ensure that all goes smoothly. They take care of the recipients from the moment they register for an organ transplant and put their name on a waiting list through to their time as outpatients after the surgery. They are often saddened or dismayed by the human relationship problems they encounter within families involved in live organ transplants but they admire organ donation and the donors who save patients with their "gift of life." Most recipient coordinators in hospitals are registered nurses and take care of both recipient candidates and recipients, especially their mental and pastoral care.

5. Donor Coordinators

Donor coordinators have no opportunity to meet the recipients and their work starts after the donor's brain death, so they frequently have complex feelings toward organ transplantation from brain-dead donors. They often ask themselves whether it is an acceptable procedure or not as a human being, although they greatly admire donor families as well as the donors themselves for what they do. They also have no opportunity to see successful recipients after organ transplantation to witness the positive fruits of their labor. All the informants I interviewed had given up their roles as donor coordinators during my research and one of them described it as a "scary job."

CRUEL MEDICAL CARE: HARVESTING ORGANS

Japanese transplant surgeons for all varieties of organ and their coordinators feel that organ transplantation can be a cruel medical treatment for

many reasons strongly connected with traditional beliefs and culture
even in modern Japan. Nevertheless, their positions toward the degree of
cruelty they envisage in organ harvesting vary according to the kinds of
organs they deal with. In addition, while remarkable improvements have
been brought to some patients' health as a result of organ transplantation
medical care, other new problems have also arisen as (often unexpected)
side-effects, including medical, social, and psychological issues, for all
concerned parties. One of these concerns the effects on surgeons of organ
harvesting: of apparently ending the life of one patient in order to save
another.

1. Heart Transplant Surgeons

Heart transplant surgeons have to harvest beating hearts from brain-
dead patients. This is an incredibly difficult procedure for them, both
practically and emotionally; they cannot help feeling guilty about the
donors, even though they are already brain-dead. As a result, they have
to alter their perspective, and try to shift their thoughts from the donors
to the recipients, attempting wholly to focus on saving the recipients'
lives because a brain-dead donor is legally dead in Japan. They cannot
help, however, being aware of the procedure they are performing and of
the fact that they have stopped a donor's heart with their own hand.

2. Liver Transplant Surgeons

Liver transplantation also usually relies on brain-dead donors, although as transplantation technology develops it is also possible from
living donors. Japan is facing a severe organ shortage and the situation
surrounding overseas transplantation is perceived as more and more difficult (Yasuoka 2010). As a result, although liver transplant surgeons
have concerns about the effects of the harvesting procedure on living
donors, they recommend organ transplantation from a living donor in
the family circle where possible to increase the potential number of donated organs for their patients. The choice of family donor is also, however, a fraught decision. First, the operation is very difficult and gives rise
to a number of risks, not only in harvesting the organ but also in transplanting the liver. In some cases liver recipients have died after organ
donation from a family member: how likely is someone to donate their
organ to a member of their family when there is a risk of death? Second,
sometimes a family member cannot donate an organ—this removes the
hope of organ transplantation from both potential donor and recipient.
For these reasons among others, future donors have to undergo counsel-
ing from psychiatrists. All these problems surrounding organ donation
within the family circle are cruel elements for liver transplant surgeons.

3. Kidney Transplant Surgeons

Kidney transplant surgeons are different from heart and liver transplant surgeons in that kidney transplantation has become a relatively common medical treatment, although it is not a simple procedure and there is a severe worldwide shortage of kidneys as well as other organs. As mentioned earlier, kidney failure patients have a wider range of alternative options than recipients of other organs, including brain-dead donors, heart-dead donors and living donors. Nevertheless, all recipients entrust surgeons with their lives and every case of kidney transplantation is different; for example, some recipients have only one family member, which puts additional pressure on the surgeon. A Japanese living kidney donor died recently; this case not only shocked the kidney transplant world but also had an effect on other organ transplants from living donors, as it revealed that organ donation from living donors is not entirely safe.

4. Recipient Coordinators

Recipient coordinators have to organize organ donation and reception and also frequently end up having to address inter-family issues which become bogged down with emotion. Organ transplantation from living donors within the family circle can produce very human emotional problems of ego and desire when people face such an important matter of life and death. Recipient coordinators are sometimes unable to remain outside a difficult family quarrel as donors do or do not wish to give an organ that a recipient needs. This darker aspect of the "gift of life" makes recipient coordinators feel that the medical treatment has a cruel side and that the option of organ donation within the family circle reveals human ego and selfishness and can risk breaking family ties.

5. Donor Coordinators

Donor coordinators' work starts when they are made aware of a donor's death and they have to provide information about organ donation to the donor family, which is newly grieving and often in shock. They also have no involvement with the surviving recipient, which might allow them to witness the happy result of the donation, so theirs is a really tough job. What's worse, people sometimes call their office to try to sell organs and ask the price offered, which adversely affects the coordinators' morale. Many donor coordinators who participated in interviews for this research were unavailable for follow-ups as they had quit their jobs and left the world of organ transplantation, feeling that it is a cruel business. The lack of social consensus about whether organ donation is acceptable is also a factor of the cruelty donor coordinators perceive in organ donation issues.

6. Feelings of Medical Staff toward Donors

The interview research shows that all transplant surgeons and coordinators admire organ transplantation as an innovative medical treatment, but most have complex feelings toward organ harvesting. It is a natural human reaction to hesitate to harvest organs from a recently dead body. Surgeons in particular feel guilt toward donors when they harvest organs, especially when harvesting beating hearts from brain-dead donors, although they also admire organ transplantation, and appreciate the donor and donor families. They appreciate the decisions made by the donor and donor family and feel a strong weight of responsibility toward all concerned parties to ensure that the operation is a success.

7. Feelings of Medical Staff toward Donor Families

Although transplant medical staff cannot communicate with deceased donors, they can have a conversation with donor families and, according to my narrative data, many of them feel dilemmas in the course of their work. In decisions about organ donation the donor family has more control than the donor: most donors do not have or have not kept their families informed of a donation will, so organ donation is often decided by donor families during their initial sorrow at the loss of a family member. When transplant surgeons ask permission to harvest organs from a donor, they must try not to feel guilt toward the donor's family. They will inevitably feel sorry for the donor and donor family, however, since they cannot save the donor's life, and they cannot help but feel that this aspect of their job contains an element of cruelty.

THE DILEMMAS OF TRANSPLANT SURGEONS AND COORDINATORS

The transplant surgeons' narratives show that while they admire organ transplantation as the "gift of life," they feel cruel harvesting an organ from a brain-dead donor and also feel guilty taking a scalpel into a healthy body to harvest an organ from a living donor. Japanese medical professionals feel ambivalence as they face these new dilemmas created by new and emerging medical technologies with the newly created agent of the donor, whose brain function has died but whose organs are still working. As one transplant surgeon told me, "Harvesting a beating heart from a brain-dead patient gave me the illusion that I had ended the donor patient's life." This section considers some of the dilemmas faced by transplant surgeons and coordinators and the methods they use to cope with and negotiate these difficult situations.

1. Heart Transplant Surgeons

Heart transplant surgeons advocate heart donations from brain-dead patients to increase organ donation numbers for heart recipient candidates who have few chances to receive a new heart within Japan. When they have a donor they can perform a heart transplant, but to do so they have to harvest a beating heart. Recently, thanks to developments in organ preservation and improvements in methods to prepare for organ replacement, they can give more time to the bereaved family to spend the final days with the brain-dead patient. During surgery they often feel that they should be working to save the donor's life instead, but if they do not harvest the heart they cannot save the recipient, so they must force themselves to believe that brain death is actual death, and that by harvesting an organ they are saving a life.

2. Liver Transplant Surgeons

Japan faces a severe organ shortage, so liver transplant surgeons first advocate organ donation from brain-dead patients. Second, they inform potential donors about donor cards and demonstrate how to keep the completed card with the donation will. Third, they recommend overseas transplants, but only in the case of children under fifteen years old, who have almost no donors in Japan: before the Japanese organ transplantation law was revised, organ donation from children was banned. When the Japanese mass media published admiring stories about overseas transplants, the surgeons criticized this approach, because worldwide organ self-sufficiency should be the aim of every country. Because of the lack of "home-grown" donors the dilemma for liver transplant surgeons is whether or not to perform invasive organ harvesting surgery on a live donor, which is a risky procedure for both donor and recipient.

3. Kidney Transplant Surgeons

The wider variety of possible treatments for kidney recipients, even though treatment is more common as a result, gives rise to additional and different dilemmas for kidney transplant surgeons. Recipients have twice as many opportunities to receive organs because humans have two kidneys, so kidney transplant surgeons have a wider variety of recipients and may find themselves operating more than once on the same patient, since a transplanted kidney may need replacing within five to seven years. Since kidneys can be donated by living donors, this can mean that the kidney transplant surgeon has to perform an invasive operation on more than one living donor, thereby harming more than one healthy body in order to assist and give some additional life to the recipient. Japanese kidney recipients mostly depend on living donor within the family circle or overseas transplants in south Asian countries—surprisingly, numbers of kidney donations from brain-dead donors have decreased since the Japanese transplantation law was revised.

4. Recipient Coordinators

Recipient coordinators support recipients not only in the physical aspects of the transplantation procedure but also by providing mental support for a long time both before and after the operation. They are also often involved in the family issues caused by the different attitudes and expectations of the various family members when the recipients receive organs from living donors within their family circle. Some recipients and recipients' families have cultural and traditional beliefs that make them feel shame to live with another's organ. Indeed, some recipients' family members consider that organ reception is behavior that exposes someone to ridicule in Japan, especially in more traditional areas of Japan such as more westerly parts or the countryside. Recipient coordinators admire the "gift of life" because recipients can't survive without organ donation, but they prefer organ donation from brain-dead donors as they are often appalled at the problems created by living donors and their families.

5. Donor Coordinators

Donor coordinators have no opportunity to see the successful recipients, which makes theirs the toughest job in the organ transplantation world: they know only the sorrowful side of the organ transplant process, not the joyful outcome. Rumors abound in Japanese society about how donor families demand money for organs or are threatened by medical staff, but donor coordinators find that donor family members are usually mature and thoughtful people who only want to make a social contribution after their relative's death by donating their organs to offer someone life. When the coordinators receive phone calls from organ sellers asking for prices, it also makes them sad and despair of human nature. As a result of such an abundance of grief, their dilemma is that they are no longer sure whether organ transplantation is a positive medical treatment or whether it should not be used for humans because of the reactions resulting from it.

6. Harvesting Organs for Recipients

Transplant surgeons, and especially coordinators, are aware of and need to consider the dilemmas of transplant recipients concerning the harvesting of organs as they try to come to terms with the procedure. They also have to deal with significant ethical issues surrounding the harvesting of living donor's organs, since the procedure is a risky one for both the donor and the recipient, and both aspects have to be taken into consideration. According to my data, they see organ transplantation as the "gift of life" to save recipients and this phrase encourages their mission as medical specialists, except when harvesting organs. In an ideal world, they want to save both the recipients and the donors, but they try to focus on their medical mission to save the recipient without fail.

1. Organ recipients often talk about the donation will of the donor or the donor family's decision to donate an organ, but they tend not to refer to organ harvesting directly so that they do not have to consider the full practical implications of the decision to donate, while both surgeons and coordinators are very much aware of the details and requirements surrounding organ harvesting. Nevertheless, all organ recipients have great appreciation for donors and donor families.

2. There are similar issues surrounding harvesting organs from living family members. These are most often from parents for children, although because of developing technology non-blood family such as spouses can also donate, and more donors are needed because of the dire shortage of organs available in Japan. The living donor is frequently in the same family home, so relatives care equally for the donor and recipient as part of their family. Their reactions can cause family rifts that the surgeons and coordinators have to negotiate in the process of organizing the transplant operation.

3. Thanks to the development of emerging medical technology, re-transplantation is now possible and recipients (mostly kidney) can receive more than one donation so they have plural donors and donated organs. As a result, paradoxically, the organ shortage has become more and more severe as more and more organs are desperately needed. In terms of kidney transplantation, however, PET (preemptive transplantation) has shown encouraging results and recipients have good prognosis.

7. Harvesting Organs for Recipients' Families

Much attention has been given to donor families' roles in the decision to donate organs and far less to the families of recipients, but with live organ transplantation within the family circle the same people are the family of both the donor and the recipient. This can cause significant issues for transplant surgeons and coordinators as they have to negotiate the minefield of family feelings and understand the stresses of family members grappling with decisions to undergo invasive surgery to harvest organs for a family member. Different family members can hold different opinions about the appropriate course of action depending on their relationship to the donor and recipient: one side may feel a donor should donate an organ to ensure the recipient's survival while the other may feel that the potential donor should not be put at risk of medical problems themselves, which might lead to two seriously ill patients in the family. Such diversity of opinion puts severe stress and pressure on transplant surgeons and coordinators as they try to take on board both points of view and also have two lives at risk and needing to be saved.

The next section introduces Japanese transplant surgeons' and coordinators' narratives, paying attention to the specific organ of their specialism.

TRANSPLANT SURGEONS' NARRATIVES

Emerging medical technology has produced many specialist professionals to administer the new treatments. Organ transplant surgeons are a new type of specialist with a license to perform organ transplantation surgery and treatment, but there were very few transplant departments in Japanese hospitals when I first started to collect my interview research (2002–2003). Recently, some larger general hospitals have set up transplant departments or organ replacement divisions but this is not yet common. In many hospitals organ transplantation treatment falls within the remit of the department corresponding to the particular organ: heart transplantation in circulatory surgery, liver transplantation in digestive organ surgery, kidney transplantation in urinary surgery, and so on.

Japanese transplant surgeons complete their education or undertake their medical training careers in the United States before returning to Japan. Although they come from different backgrounds, their passion for organ transplantation, determination to assist recipients, and appreciation for donors are the same. Nevertheless, they experience various difficulties with the duties required by their chosen profession. Because of a lack of brain-dead or deceased donors with donation wills they have to consider harvesting organs from living donors, but it is difficult for a surgeon to be comfortable performing unnecessary surgery on a healthy body. Harvesting an organ from a brain-dead patient is also an incredibly challenging task, especially in the case of removing a still-beating heart and thereby hastening the end of a patient's life.

TRANSPLANT SURGEONS' MEDICAL ASSESSMENTS
OF ORGAN TRANSPLANTATION

The donor is a new agent created by organ transplantation technology, which transforms both the mission and the concept of life reflected in the personal philosophy of a surgeon. The process of organ transplantation from a brain-dead donor follows a medical pathway from assessing a donor to be brain-dead to harvesting their organs to transplanting the organs. Transplant surgeons give different assessments of these three elements from a medical and a personal perspective, but they admire the donor and donor family for making the decision to donate organs based on altruism. All concerned parties appear to find themselves affected by the existence of this new agent of the donor—including transplant surgeons, whose role can be seen as a mediator between donors and recipients—and feel that it has some form of control over them.

Surgeons' assessments of organ transplantation from living donors vary with their own specialties, positions, and roles, containing a mix of individual policy and traditional beliefs. Most surgeons have no alternative but to consider live organ transplants because of the lack of available donors, but their assessments are very ambiguous, complex, and confusing. When they focus on saving the recipient's life, they can consider the organ donation to be the "gift of life" and can thus appreciate the living donor, who has made the self-sacrifice. Simultaneously, however, they have many ethical and emotional difficulties, as when they accept living donors it means that they will have to insert a scalpel into a healthy body (Lock 2002).

Doctor Matsui's Assessment — "I'm Sometimes Tempted but Wouldn't Leave the Job"

Doctor Matsui[1] is forty-seven years old, married, a medical school graduate, and a transplant physician, living with his wife and two sons. He is a heart and blood vessel specialist and has been a heart transplant physician since 1997 in the United States and Japan.

> An American chief organ transplant doctor and I go out for a drink together frequently and we have lost track of the number of times we have discussed being tempted to leave this job or trying to quit organ transplant medicine because it is extremely tough, both physically and mentally. We often decide to quit the specialism, but then we encounter a dying patient who receives a transplanted organ from a donor and witness the moment the recipient is revived, against all the odds, and regains their life. This dramatic situation shows things outside our understanding, such as the great love of family or various aspects of the recipient that are revealed through organ transplantation. I think that it is the happiest moment for humans: when we look at something beautiful or good. That's why we are tempted to quit but we wouldn't, and we still keep performing organ transplantation to see the recipients' happy faces; and not only the recipients but also their families and other people involved. The chief doctor of our transplant team in the United States once told me that when we look at the recipients' smiles, they become our motivation.

This doctor is not in fact a surgeon but a transplant physician, of which there are only a few in Japan. In the United States, transplant medicine is a treatment involving extensive team work, in which many specialists come together and their roles complement each other within the organ transplant department; this is not yet the situation in Japan, where transplant sections are structured differently within various hospital departments. This doctor holds the heart transplant physician license, qualifying him to assess the organ from the donor and to perform the clinical examination of the recipient's diseased organ. Many recipient candidates visit him from all over Japan every day but only 10 percent to 12 percent of them need a heart transplant.

1. Doctor Matsui's narrative begins by discussing the harshness of organ transplantation, showing how both Japanese and American transplant medical staff feel that it is a difficult line of work, to the extent that even the chief of transplantation surgery considers quitting. But it ends by emphasizing the wonderfulness of the treatment, showing the ambivalent feelings created for all working in the field. His attitude toward his patients is very tender but he tries to be strict with himself and use his strong will to manage his feelings of guilt.

2. Doctors have mixed emotions toward heart transplantation from brain-dead donors, although they chose to train for and practice their job, while recipients and donors (and donor families) cannot choose their destiny for organ transplantation. Some heart transplant surgeons feel the unfairness of having to be a concerned party, because it is nobody's choice to be a brain-dead donor or a heart recipient, but the heart transplant surgeon can only save the recipient and not the donor.

3. Although people say that Japanese organ donation numbers are the lowest and American numbers are the highest in the world because of the spirit of the "gift of life," this narrative shows the American and Japanese transplant staff sharing their mixed feelings over a drink and chat, emphasizing that the organ donation number and the nationality do not necessarily correspond.

This is the only narrative data from a transplant physician in Japan (there are both transplant surgeons and transplant physicians only in the United States and a few other developed countries). The next five narratives come from transplant surgeons, enabling comparison of the characteristic differences between the professions, although all are Japanese medical doctors.

Surgeon Kawasaki's Assessment — "Involvement in Revivifying Medical Treatment"

Surgeon Kawasaki is forty-seven years old, married, a medical school graduate (PhD), and a transplant surgeon (urological surgery), living with his wife and mother. He is a kidney and urinary organs expert, particularly specializing in kidney dysfunction and transplantation, and has been a kidney transplant surgeon since 1983 in the United States and Japan.

> I think that organ transplantation such as liver, heart and kidney transplants offers fantastic treatment. I truly feel so, and would describe it with one simple word: "Excellent." When a child who might die is in my care, if he/she is unlucky I have to continue ordinary treatment without an organ transplant. However, when a new organ is transplanted in the child's body and treatment is maintained, he/she becomes suddenly revitalized and able to live a long time. I have the impression that organ transplantation is very close to reviving medical treatment. That's why I was motivated to be a transplant surgeon. It was at the time when cyclosporine was introduced and the survival rate was increasing rapidly. Seeing a successful kidney recipient was such a strong impact for me: I thought, "Oh, organ recipients can survive," and I decided I wanted to be a transplant surgeon as I thought that transplant treatment was so great.

Surgeon Aoki's Assessment — "Organ and Tissue Donation: The Only Cost Is a Little Love"

Surgeon Aoki is forty-six years old, married, a medical school graduate, medical doctor, and university instructor, living with his wife and four sons. He is a kidney, pancreas, and liver transplantation specialist and has been a transplant surgeon since 1982 in the United States (two years) and Japan.

> I think that organ donation from a dead person is a wonderful thing. In fact, I see many patients, and I know plenty of very happy recipients who I have treated with organ transplantation. . . . There are many recipients whose organs I checked myself, then I personally harvested organs from dead bodies and transplanted the donors' organs into the recipients, after which they survived and left the hospital. I think that the wonder of organ transplantation is felt most by transplant surgeons: we feel best ourselves how admirable a treatment it is. One of the most important things for me, through my experience of organ transplant procedures over the years, is knowing that organ transplantation is the most fantastic treatment I've ever performed. . . . I've seen hundreds of recipients go through the process from the start of treatment to the present day: before organ transplantation, undergoing transplant surgery, and after the organs are transplanted and they have survived and become revitalized. I see my patients, made recipients by

my surgery. I have really come to understand the excellence of organ transplantation. However, the focus of all my thankfulness is organ donation by donors and donor families. I really feel the warmth of the donor's organ donation and the donor family's decision to donate their family member's organ. I really, really appreciate them from the bottom of my heart. . . . I like this phrase: "organ and tissue donation: the only cost is a little love."

Surgeon Sasaki's Assessment — "Offering a 'Gift of Life' Just Like a Buddha"

Surgeon Sasaki is sixty-nine years old, married, a medical school graduate, and a medical doctor, living with his wife and two children. He is a kidney specialist and has been a kidney transplant surgeon since 1968 in Japan.

> The "gift of life," how should I say . . . is one of the behavioral principles that makes the world turn: one of the most important. Such a concept: it is a truly wonderful, brilliant jewel for human society to have such concepts as the "gift of life." If we didn't have the medical treatment of organ transplantation, the "gift of life" itself would not exist. It is completely different from curing patients with medicines or operations. It's a jewel, isn't it? We should feel selfless love. The donor's bereaved family members, whose relative suffered an accidental death or death by disease, transform from an ordinary bereaved family to gradually become a donor family, don't they? . . . They are a cast as avuncular as a Buddha. The donor family can approach organ donation with gracious human love. . . . So giving the "gift of life" is like a Buddha's giving.

These narratives from a heart transplant physician, a liver transplant surgeon, and two kidney transplant surgeons describe the wonderfulness and attractiveness of organ transplantation. Their admiration is first for the results of organ transplantation for recipients of all types of organs and the new lease of life: it gives their patients a miraculous treatment. Second, they admire both the concept and the behavior created by organ donation among donors and donor families, in which the acts of all the agents are based on altruism. They have differing degrees of admiration for the altruism of donor families, depending on their motivation for the donation; nevertheless, they notice the maturing process experienced, whatever the original motivation, as the family progresses from a bereaved to a donor family.

1. Cyclosporine, which was discovered when Surgeon Kawasaki was a medical school student, significantly raised the survival rate of kidney organ recipients in the 1980s. He was stunned by the improved results, seeing them as almost miraculous, and this became his motivation to become a transplant surgeon to provide transplantation treatment. However, he had many complaints about the

Japanese medical world compared to his experience in the United States, such as the overall closed medical society, which combines the old-fashioned hierarchical world with modern innovation and financial problems (including low salaries for transplant surgeons, who still take on a great deal of voluntary work to promote organ donation and transplantation). He added that the "gift of life" has two interpretations: the narrow sense focuses on donating an organ, while the broader sense concerns supplying a whole better quality of life.

2. Surgeon Aoki has an addictive pace of work, taking charge of both organ harvesting from donors and organ transplantation for recipients, working with patients continuously before, during, and after surgery. He is proud of being an organ transplant surgeon and very satisfied with the survival of his organ recipients, although his strongest appreciation is for organ donors and their families. He criticized the attitude of the Japanese mass media to recipients, however, saying that news stories focus on charitable overseas transplants that save Japanese babies, not mentioning that if a Japanese baby receives an organ in Australia then an Australian baby may die instead. He felt that the media instead should shed light on the donor families as well as the recipients, and should advocate organ donation and making clear donation wills to improve the situation in the country. He was also concerned that the media watch transplant surgeons to try to uncover any mistakes that they can link back to the infamous "Wada case" for the sake of a story.

3. Surgeon Sasaki is from a different generation from the other doctors: he was a pioneer of kidney transplantation in 1968 when the first heart transplant from a brain-dead donor was performed in Japan by Dr. Wada. He knows all the traumatic history of Japanese organ transplantation and he was attacked by both anti-organ transplant and anti-brain-death groups. He feels concerned at what he sees as the selfishness of people—even organ recipients themselves—who are not prepared to offer to donate their organs to help someone else to live, but he admires the concept of the "gift of life" as a Buddhist ethic.

Surgeon Tanaka's Assessment—"It Is Cruel Medical Treatment"

Surgeon Tanaka is forty-six years old, married, a medical school graduate, and a medical doctor, living with his wife, son, and daughter. He is a heart specialist and has been a heart transplant surgeon since 1983, holding a research post from 1983 to 1991, working in an overseas hospital since 1991 and registered to perform organ transplantation from brain-dead donors since 1997.

An organ harvest surgeon sees the medical record and the evidence of the life of the donor when examining the brain-dead body, having received a donation will. If the patient has brain-dead status he/she has already died under Japanese law. However, when medical doctors see the dying person, we can't abandon the feeling that we want to save him/her. We can see that the patient's heart is still beating and we are torn between trying to save the patient on the table and trying to harvest their organ to save a recipient. I can save one person by transplanting organs, and although I'm very happy to be able to save them, I have to feel sad to lose someone else. I know the patient's history, and when I give him/her preoperative sterilization and lay a cover sheet over the body, then harvest a beating heart myself, I have a feeling of bringing an end to the person' s life with my own hand. In the United States one transplant surgeon harvests the heart from a small section of the patient's chest visible under a sheet, while another implants the organ in the recipient; in Japan the same surgeon completes both parts of the process, giving the complex inhuman impression of killing one patient to save another. You see what I mean? That's why I think that organ transplantation is cruel medical treatment for transplant surgeons. . . . Well, all in all, it is painful, you understand?

Surgeon Hasegawa's Assessment — "Undertaking Pressurized Medical Treatment"

Surgeon Hasegawa is fifty years old, married, a medical school graduate, and a kidney transplant surgeon (urology), living with his wife, son, and daughter. He is a kidney specialist and has been a kidney transplant surgeon since 1980.

There is a patient in front of me, whom I know well and have treated since childhood: she is now a twenty-year-old. If she remains on dialysis she might have complications from arteriosclerosis when she is forty. What is more, she can only hope for a kidney donation from her mother, not her father, because he has other complications so her options are limited. I must try to arrange a successful kidney transplant, but I can't help avoiding emotional expectations. As surgeons our feelings are often mixed and we feel torn over some decisions we have to make, but I try to maintain a calm professional outlook and give that impression to others. My patients take a serious view of my attitude and it can affect them. There is particular pressure on us when performing children's transplant surgery. I try to be objective, but it is a very difficult thing to do: it is a hard task for us transplant surgeons. People say that kidney transplantation is not as great a risk to the recipient's life as heart transplant and liver transplant surgery. A kidney transplant contributes to raising the quality of life of a recipient rather than saving a life, but it does in fact risk the recipient's life, even though to a lesser extent; as does any surgery.

These two surgeons, one a heart transplant surgeon and the other a kidney transplant surgeon, offer very different assessments especially for organ transplant surgery processes (harvesting and transplanting organs). Heart and liver transplantation risks the recipient's life as a medical treatment but kidney transplantation is less of a risk to life (although there is still an element of risk with any operation), instead contributing to raising the recipient's quality of life. There are also differences in donor availability: heart transplants rely on only brain-dead donors, but kidney donors can be living donors as well as dead donors (both brain-dead and heart-dead). This means that these two transplant surgeons have very different perceptions of the level of cruelty of organ transplantation.

This comparison of surgeons' narratives is very rare and precious because most people make the mistake of thinking that all transplant surgeons are the same, regardless the kinds of organs. According to the narrative data, the depth of cruelty of organ transplantation is perceived differently depending on the organ specialism of the transplant surgeon, as well as the individual personality. The heart transplant surgeon feels the cruelty of harvesting a beating heart from a brain-dead donor but the kidney transplant surgeon feels pressure from both the recipient and the living donor in the family circle. In sum, transplant surgeons narrated that harvesting organs puts them under great pressure mentally and technically from all kinds of donors, whether brain-dead, heart-dead, or living donors.

Recipient Coordinator Morita's Assessment— "Organ Donation in Japan is about Taking, Not Giving"

Recipient coordinator Morita is thirty-five years old, single, and a university graduate, living alone. She is a liver specialist and has been a recipient coordinator since 1993.

> I thought that organ transplantation was wonderful when I saw a living child revitalized by a liver transplant. I had seen many children pass away with yellow shins caused by bi-biliary atresia, their bellies swollen with hepatic cirrhosis, then reduced to skin and bone. When I see a living liver transplant, it is performed by harming a living donor, isn't it? For parents, if their child might die, they think that they must try to do something to save them, but although they are happy to accept an organ they often refuse to agree to donate their and their families' organs. If your brother or sister needs a liver, they really want you to donate for them from the heart. There are children who donate their organs to their parents. If they say "I want to give my liver to my brother/sister," I wonder whether they are perfectly serious and have thought about their future before deciding on organ donation. When they think about the possibility of the organ donor having a risk of death it sometimes happens that they might decide against donating the organ or not find a living organ transplant available in the family

circle. There is even just the option to decide for organ donation or against. . . . Once a living donor candidate decides against organ donation, the relationship between the donor and the recipient becomes worse within the family circle. I don't think that living transplantation is a good thing like organ donation. But there is no choice, given the restrictions of current medical technology.

Recipient Coordinator Toyota's Assessment—"An Opportunity to Consider Life and Death"

Recipient coordinator Toyota is thirty-five years old, single, a nursing school graduate, and university student (via a correspondence course), living alone. She is a heart, lung, pancreas, liver, and kidney specialist and has been a recipient coordinator since 2001.

> I think that organ transplantation has become an opportunity for Japanese people to think about many things. Considering the issue of brain death is a good opportunity for me to think about my own death. Considering the issue of living donors is also a chance to think about organ donation from a healthy person, hurting his/her body, and even relatives. For a recipient . . . the process of organ transplantation allows them to think about life and death from organ donation to organ reception. I think that for Japanese people there is no chance to think over and over about life and death, so it has become a good motivation: I think that it's a good thing. We Japanese had no chance to think "What is death?" when growing up. Suddenly, when told "Let's think about death," we can't think about it. When we are school age, we have very little chance to think about death. . . . In my own case I had no opportunity.

Donor Coordinator Matsushita's Assessment—"It Is a Scary Job"

Donor coordinator Matsushita is thirty-five years old, single, a college graduate, and nurse, living with her parents, brother, and sister. She has been a donor coordinator since 2000.

> My opinion of transplant medicine has changed entirely. I thought that organ transplantation was a simple treatment. I couldn't imagine at all that it was a medical treatment with such a strong social aspect. I thought that it was enough that a person wanted to donate his/her organs and another person wanted to receive someone's organ, and their wishes would both come true. . . . I thought that organ transplantation was a noble medical treatment, but it isn't: there are pros and cons. I have had many bitter experiences in the job. Before I became a coordinator I thought that my role was to make the donor's donation will and the recipient's wish to receive an organ come true, but things were not so simple. In reality many obstacles stand in the way of both sides of the process of making these wishes come true. I encountered so many bad things (such as selling or stealing organs, murders and kid-

nappings, or painful inter-familial fighting and rifts) that it is very difficult for me to understand whether this medical transplantation is in fact good or bad for humans. It causes very deep philosophical and ethical problems, and the more I learn about it the more I realize how naïve I was when I began the job. There is a very dark side to the world of organ transplantation, which scares me greatly.

These three coordinators' narratives describe the difficulties surrounding organ transplantation issues, with different points of views depending on their position as recipient or donor coordinators. A kidney transplant surgeon once advised me that "[n]obody can understand the issues of organ transplantation without coordinators." After these interviews both the recipient and donor coordinators faced very tough problems: their work is much more important and difficult than I had imagined. In fact, while all the coordinators I interviewed were lovely people, since the original interviews all have quit their roles and left the organ transplant world. It seems that their responsibilities were too great and they became worn out both physically and mentally. It is important that the organ transplant network should also pay attention to the physical and mental health of transplant medical staff.

1. Recipient coordinator Morita is a nurse and trained to be a recipient coordinator in Australia. She is considered a pioneer in the field of recipient coordination in Japan. She understands the full situation surrounding organ recipients' matters in both a positive and a negative way—she knows more than transplant surgeons in some ways. She values organ transplantation as one of the emerging medical technologies and understands that organ donation depends on precious human love that supports transplantation, but she has been utterly disgusted by the troubles and problems she has encountered surrounding living transplants, especially inter-family quarrels.

2. Recipient coordinator Toyota is also a nurse but her role as a coordinator is different from Morita's, who trained for her license in Australia when there was as yet no such system in Japan, because it was before the original organ transplantation law was implemented. After the law come into force many hospitals needed recipient coordinators: Toyota works in a hospital but is also studying with a Japanese university to get her license via a correspondence course. While Morita is a specialist in liver transplants, Toyota works with various organs; thus, their impressions of organ transplantation are different. Toyota's views are more neutral and she advocates thinking about life and death more deeply.

3. Donor coordinator Matsushita is also a nurse but her role as a donor coordinator shows the opposite side of the process from that experienced by the recipient coordinators. There are very few do-

nor coordinators so it is very difficult for researchers to contact them. It is quite easy to find a recipient coordinator in a hospital, while a donor coordinator's workplace is often unknown. Matsushita described her job as "scary," indicating the various issues she has encountered throughout the phases of organ transplantation such as harvesting, receiving, and replacing the organ. The agents she deals with as part of the job include donors, recipients, donor families, and recipient families (living donors in the family circle). In her attitude toward organ transplantation she absolutely respects concerned parties' different values of life and death, feeling that all should be entitled to their views. However, she wonders whether organ transplant treatment is good medical care for human beings. Unfortunately, she quit her donor coordinator job after the interview, so it is impossible to undertake follow-up research with her. The high job turnover rate also shows how "scary" the job of donor coordinator is.

4. These different professionals' interpretations of organ transplantation also vary, depending on whether they are a recipient or a donor coordinator. Recipient coordinators advocate organ transplantation from brain-dead donors but not living donors because of the battles this can cause within the family. The donor coordinator was unnerved by the numerous issues she discovered surrounding organ transplantation and felt she was walking into a labyrinth of problems. Their different attitudes shed light on our views as we think about this medical treatment.

It is hard to generalize about transplant medical professionals' attitudes toward organ transplantation because each specialty is different, reflecting deep but varied concepts of life and death. In Japan people are generally not interested in organ transplantation issues but are concerned parties and consider them strongly and repeatedly; this makes them think about their whole life philosophies. It is important for non-concerned parties to understand that organ transplantation is not a simple treatment and has wider philosophical ramifications.

According to the narrative data, organ transplantation is strengthened and developed by each transplant surgeon's and each coordinator's professional skills and their own personality characteristics. Japanese transplant surgeons have to transform their traditional ideas about the relationship between a doctor and patient in a revolutionary way, moving from a paternalistic to a mediating role, and organ transplantation sets very tough challenges for donors, donor families, and recipients, who cannot be passive recipients of medical treatment but must make difficult decisions.

Organ transplantation stimulates the most troubling aspects of human beings' attitudes to life and death: saving a recipient is an important and rewarding event for everyone concerned, but someone's death (including brain death) is something to be hoped against, that we try to avoid and hide from—a sad event. However, the essence of organ transplantation reveals the essence of life and death clearly, as one person's death supports another's life. All the concerned parties narrate their own various interpretations, and everyone has been through the mental process over and over to reach a rational conclusion that they construct themselves. Most people when thinking about organ transplantation are interested in the organ recipients and donors but not so much in the transplant surgeons and coordinators, but these medical professionals' interactions with the recipients and donor families are the most important element of the process and worth considerable new research. Transplant surgeons and transplant physicians offer different assessments of organ transplantation, as do heart, liver, and kidney transplant surgeons, as well as recipient and donor coordinators, each informed by their different roles and experiences.

"MEDIATED LIFE"

"Transplanted life" is a term coined by a heart transplant surgeon in Japan who harvests hearts from brain-dead donors, but who is highly conscious of the cruelty of the procedure and thus tries to shift his feelings from considering the donor to focusing on his mission to save the heart recipient. Organ transplantation is called the "big bang" or "mushroom cloud" of medical treatment in Japanese medical society because of the immense changes it has brought about. The Japanese medical world has had to change as a result of organ transplantation from brain-dead donors, especially in its traditional doctor–patient relationship. The traditional and historic paternalistic Japanese relationship between medical doctors and patients is very strong, but organ transplant doctors have to beg for organ donations from donor families, setting aside their paternalistic attitudes and power and becoming "mediators." As a result, "mediated life" is the new term used by transplant medical staff for their changed relationship with their patients. In the course of my research I got the impression that transplant medical professionals were completely different from other medical doctors. All the transplant surgeons and coordinators I met were very modest and defy the arrogant stereotype of Japanese medical professionals. They have a unique and special passion for organ transplantation surgery and share something in common in their minds and behaviors, which we can discover through their narratives.

The number of transplant surgeons accounts for only a small percentage of the total number of medical doctors in Japan, but the mediating attitude of the few and the paternalistic attitude of the many are completely different—almost opposites. It is difficult to understand how transplant surgeons, who are required to have paternalistic attitudes as surgeons to perform successful medical treatment, in fact become mediators. Organ transplantation cannot start without an organ donation from a donor and the essential requirements for this are a donation will and the joint decision making of donor families. Transplant surgeons have to enlist cooperation from both the donor and the donor family, and must thus change their attitude from paternalism to mediating between the donor's human love and the recipient's wish to survive, as a sacred calling. According to my data, transplant surgeons feel delighted to save a recipient with a donated organ, and appreciate and admire the decision to donate an organ, but they feel a kind of guilt toward the donors for harvesting their organs (Yasuoka 2013). Surgeons feel that organ transplantation is a wonderful treatment, but organ harvesting is a medical procedure that causes them difficulties (Starzl 1992).

NOTES

1. All names (of transplant surgeons and coordinators, recipients, and donor families) used in the text are pseudonyms.

REFERENCES

Inhorn, M., and Wentzell, E. (2011). "Embodying Emergent Masculinities: Reproductive and Sexual Health Technologies in the Middle East and Mexico." *American Ethnologist* 38(4): 801–815.

Lock, M. (2002). *Twice Dead: Organ Transplants and the Reinvention of Death*. Berkeley: University of California Press.

Starzl, T. (1992). *The Puzzle People: Memories of a Transplant Surgeon*. Pittsburgh: University of Pittsburgh Press.

Yasuoka, M. K. (2006). "Rebirthable Life: Medical Anthropology Study of the Concept of Life according to Concerned Parties Involved in Brain Death and Organ Transplantation." PhD thesis: Department of History and Anthropology (Medical Anthropology), Graduate School of Letters, Hokkaido University, Sapporo, Japan (unpublished).

———. (2010). "Medical Refugees in Japan: From Overseas Transplants to Organ Self-Sufficiency for Japanese Recipients." *Applied Ethics: Challenges for the 21st Century*, 85–97. Sapporo, Japan: Center for Applied Ethics and Philosophy, Hokkaido University.

———. (2013). "Rebirthable Life: Narratives and Reproductive Life of Japanese Brain-Dead Donors." *Research Journal of Graduate Students of Letters* (Japan) 8: 73–81.

THREE
Narratives of Recipients

INTRODUCTION

To be honest, there was no space to think about organ reception or anything else. I mean there was not only no physical space in terms of time but also no mental and emotional space. Because of expected events I was totally upset by more than the burden of my illness. It was a Saturday and my dialysis treatment was over. I came home; it was an extremely cold day, almost snowing, and my house was empty as my family was out. When I got home I first turned on the heater in my room, and as I was giving a sigh of relief, I got a phone call. This came without any warning: it was so unexpected and sudden that, all in all, I was too upset psychologically to think about the future. Really, I was in no condition to think about my future after organ reception or anything like that. —An organ recipient's narrative

Successful organ reception is the highlight of the organ transplantation process, resulting in the recipient's happiness, better health, and appreciation for donors and donor families. Outside pregnancy, there is no other medical situation in which a body can maintain the vital activities of another person's organs, and this developing medical technology can be seen as a kind of miracle. Both the quality of life of recipients and the overall assessment of a transplant are influenced by many factors, however, including the specifics of the organ, the recipient, his or her disease and medical condition, and the status of the donor (whether brain-dead, heart-dead, or living). This chapter introduces a number of narratives from organ recipients.

All parties are grateful for organ donations, whether from brain-dead, heart-dead, or living donors, from within Japan or overseas (the United States and Australia). Most recipients are happy to receive organs and go on to live fulfilling lives, advocating organ transplantation all over the world as a result of their own experiences, but not all of them. There are many elements of the organ donation process that only recipients themselves may recognize and be able to share with others, having survived transplantation through the use of immunosuppressant drugs. Although organ transplantation is not an easy medical treatment, the recipients in the main represent the positive aspects of the light and dark sides of the emerging medical technology.

Nevertheless, tracing the diversity not only of the happiness felt but also of the difficulties faced by recipients is also important in order to understand the darker side of organ transplantation. As seen through their narratives, the range of emotions they battle with—from a ray of hope to fear of the transplant failing, and from happiness and appreciation of the donor's organ to guilt at the donor's death—should not be ignored. Many recipients feel guilty because a donor died and in order for them to be alive now: this means that recipients' present life is founded on the ultimate sacrifice of donors. The recipients' experiences of the "gift of life" are a useful textbook that can help others to understand organ transplantation. Unfortunately, these narratives are extremely rare for three reasons.

1. Emerging medical technology has produced a number of new agents, including both donors and recipients (of both organs and blood transfusions).
2. Organ transplantation requires anonymity except in the case of the "thank you letter" from recipient to donor, so it is difficult to identify and find recipients and undertake formal recorded interviews. I was told by both fellow anthropologists and medical staff when I started my research that I would find it very difficult to set up interviews with concerned parties.
3. Organ donation numbers in Japan are the lowest in the world and the Japanese organ shortage is the most severe. As a result, most recipients rely on living or overseas donors, which makes finding these recipients even more difficult as they may not be on hospital waiting lists or belong to organ donor organizations as they may feel their actions shameful, making their narrative data both extremely rare and particularly valuable (Yasuoka 2006).

RECIPIENTS' REACTIONS TO ORGAN RECEPTION AND DONORS

Recipients hope for a bright future with the "gift of life" of a donated organ, hoping that they will not suffer from organ rejection. Most, however, feel guilty because they recognize that they were waiting for a human organ to give them life: as a result, they also were waiting for someone's death.

Recipients undergo a variety of emotions, not only toward the donors themselves but also toward the bereaved donor families. Recipients of organs from living donors within their family also find it difficult to express their gratitude and may also feel that they are under constant surveillance for their health to ensure that they are "taking care of" the kidney from the family member. As retransplantation becomes more common, recipients may find that they owe gratitude to more than one family member and this makes the inter-family relationships even more difficult. Recipients from deceased donors appreciate the donations but do not know how to show their gratitude: while they feel that they cannot offer enough thanks for the "gift of life" senders, they are simultaneously concerned to avoid hurting the feelings of grieving donor families. Many recipients would like to write a letter of thanks to show their appreciation but do not know how best to express their feelings and how to address the donor family with tact and sensitivity. Some recipients believe that the donor family must be happy as well as the recipient (and his/her family), and say "Thank you!" innocently; some recipients suspect donor families' sadness and are more tentative.

The recipients' narratives show that three important factors have great influence over their lives after organ reception—their gratitude for the donor's organ (sometimes including gratitude for the donor family's part in the organ donation decision-making process), their wish to offer some form of reciprocation to the bereaved family, and their feelings of guilt toward the donor and donor family. In general, recipients do not feel particularly aware of their role as part of a chain of events in the organ transplantation process until after the event. Most recipients are advised to undergo organ transplant surgery by their doctors, at which stage their primary concern is for the effect of this treatment on their condition, and they give consent for surgery without necessarily considering any other parties involved. Waiting for a suitable organ is just one aspect of a series of treatments from their doctors including medication, injections, and other remedies. At this stage, recipients are primarily thinking about their own life and death: they have no particular awareness of donors and donor families. It is only after the successful organ transplant, once they have survived the operation and recuperated and are able to return to an almost normal life, that they begin to think about the donor's death and the donor family's brave decision to donate their dead family member's organ. Now the recipients feel guilty because they have survived as a result of the donor's organ but the donor is no longer alive. Finally, they start to think about offering some sort of reciprocation for the donated organ to the donor's bereaved family.

REASONS FOR AGREEING TO ORGAN RECEPTION

The relationship between surgeon and patient in Japan still tends to be a strongly paternalistic one, which means that a surgeon's recommendation is the main reason a recipient will agree to organ transplant surgery, although other factors may also have a lesser impact on the decision-making process. Many recipients are too afraid of their doctors to turn down offers of organ transplant medical treatment, and recipients and their families face various barriers concerning organ reception.

1. Doctor's Recommendation

The majority of recipients agree to organ transplantation on a surgeon's recommendation (patients do not know whether an organ transplant is needed by themselves). While informed consent is necessary for any operation, such a cutting-edge treatment requires a high level of specific medical knowledge, so most recipients have to depend on a doctor's medical opinion, although luck also plays a part in whether a matching organ becomes available. Because of the historically paternalistic relationship between Japanese patients and doctors it is rare for a recipient to refuse transplant surgery recommended by a medical professional.

2. Parents' Financial Decision

Organ transplant surgery requires a great deal of money from recipients, especially in the case of overseas transplants, and many younger recipients depend on their parents for funds because they cannot work because of their serious medical condition. If their doctor recommends an overseas transplant, some younger recipients with financial difficulties refuse, feeling that they cannot ask their parents for the price of about 200 million Yen (2 million USD). (These young recipients are generally over twenty years old, as parents will usually make decisions on behalf of recipients under the age of nineteen in Japan.) In such a case, the doctor may inform the patient's parents directly and the parents may decide to pay for an overseas transplant to save their child, but it is not easy to raise this amount and to decide to live in the United States or Australia while awaiting a donation.

3. Mother's Decision

Japanese patients under the age of sixteen usually go to a hospital pediatrics department with their mothers. The pediatrician talks to the mother about the child and they decide on a treatment plan together; the mother then explains to her husband at home, but the child is rarely involved in the decision-making process. Japanese children's rights to self-determination as patients are transferred to their mothers; hence, child recipients have their organ transplant surgery decided by their mothers.

4. Recipient's Friend's Recommendation

Doctors do not usually recommend an overseas kidney transplant because brain-dead, heart-dead, and living donors are available within Japan, but kidney failure patients usually need dialysis three days per week, during which they chat with other patients and friends and exchange their own information about overseas kidney transplantation. They may get to know someone who is able to introduce his/her transplant surgeon in the United States. However, since the World Health Organization (WHO) called for "organ self-sufficiency" in each nation, Japanese recipients have no or few chances for overseas transplants. A few recipient candidates try in secret or consider "organ tourism," attempting to buy an organ from a developing country where there is a trade in such things; this continues to cause worldwide ethical problems and to harm human rights.

6. Recipient's Wish

Most recipients are hesitant to agree to organ reception because of the many obstacles on the route to transplant surgery, although of course they want improve their health. Some recipients recognize that organ transplantation is their only real alternative; they have no hesitation in voicing their demands and they receive organs eagerly. They also believe that donor families are happy that their family member's organs should be donated.

FACTORS AFFECTING RECIPIENTS' DECISIONS

Many factors also affect the process of deciding to receive organs from donors in Japan or overseas.

1. Speed Is of the Essence When a Donor Is Found

Some recipients need an organ, such as heart, liver, or pancreas, from a brain-dead donor, but Japanese organ donation numbers are still very low and there are not enough organs available for the number of candidate recipients in need. Most are undergoing daily medical treatment while on an organ donation waiting list for an extremely long time, but once a donor is found the operation must be performed very quickly and there is no time to think about surrounding issues. As a result, the time from the initial telephone call offering the organ to waking up in recovery after surgery passes in a blur: most recipients remember very little about the organ transplant process. Many recipients told me, "Once started, everything goes too quickly for the recipient to remember, and it seems to be like watching a film at a distance."

2. Overseas Transplantation — A Range of Difficulties

Many difficulties face patients who cannot receive organ transplant surgery in Japan and have to try overseas transplantation. First, although Japan has one of the best universal health care systems in the world, this is exclusive to Japan and overseas medical costs must be paid for by patients. Most Japanese patients have to rely on street donations to collect millions of dollars for the surgery, although some rich recipients can benefit from the chance of overseas transplantation by using their own money (usually secretly). Second, recipients have a variety of different medical issues, such as the particular organ or disease involved in their illness, and the expenses covered by health insurance likewise vary according to the issue. This means that some organs and diseases are entirely covered by national health insurance, but some have lower or even no coverage, so recipients have to pay — possibly a large sum of money. For example, liver hepatitis and cirrhosis have different proportions of coverage by health insurance companies. In addition, many patients will face cultural problems, language barriers and similar when trying to travel and arrange medical care abroad (Yasuoka 2010).

3. Japanese Room — A One-in-Eight Chance of Survival

Under the original organ transplantation law (1997–2010), children under fifteen years old were banned from donating organs. It was thus very difficult for a child to receive a suitable donation in Japan, so most child liver recipients had to depend on overseas transplants. This might, of course, not lead to success, and the wait for the Japanese child in an overseas hospital could itself prove distressing. One Australian hospital, for example, had a room containing eight Japanese children waiting for organ donations. However, even Australia has an organ shortage and only one lucky Japanese child was able to receive a liver and survive. This girl recipient has since grown up in Japan, but despite being the lucky candidate, the loss of her friends on the ward made it a tough situation and she felt it as an incredibly traumatic experience and has struggled to recover from the event.

4. Waiting for Someone's Death in the United States

Some recipients go to the United States and hope that a suitable organ will become available. American hospitals have a system whereby they accept 5 percent of their patients from developing countries where healthcare provision may be low, but this 5 percent can be made up entirely of Japanese patients, and others are sent back to Japan, where there are many hospitals and appropriate levels of expertise available. When they return to Japan after successful organ transplant surgery, however, they are driven by a kind of guilt from spending that time waiting for someone's death in order to receive the organ. They also feel guilty that they are a Japanese recipient of an American organ, and feel they have to hide their race, nationality, and similar when they write a thank you letter to the donor family rather than thanking them directly. They feel that the donor family might only want their loved one's organs to go to someone of a similar background. There are insurmountable disparities between the "gift of life" givers and receivers.

5. Preparing for Death

Most kidney recipients live on dialysis to keep them alive while waiting for an organ donation, but dialysis is not as perfect an artificial organ as people may believe. Some may have to wait more than ten years, commuting for dialysis every other day without fail. In addition, there are various side effects and the longer a recipient candidate has dialysis, the more serious the likely side effects. During this time they will see many of their fellow dialysis patients die, and they can often feel that their turn is next. In one case the patient suffered from severe depression and prepared for what he felt was his own imminent death; he had no hope and could think about nothing but his impending death, gradually losing various physical abilities during the dialysis process, until in the end he took a final chance and opted for overseas transplantation.

6. No Time to Consider

Some recipients need an organ transplant when they have children of school age. The biggest factor motivating them for organ transplantation is thus their children rather than themselves. They often say "I can't die until our children grow up," or "Now I can die anytime because our sons and daughters are over twenty." Japanese recipients with children feel they do not have time to consider their own lives and choose organ reception because of their family circumstances, without a great deal of consideration.

7. Requiring a Second Organ Donation

The more organ transplantation becomes a regular medical treatment, the more complex, diverse, and serious the processes faced by recipients become. Many recipients expected rose-tinted lives after organ transplantation, but unfortunately the donated organ cannot work forever. Kidney recipients may have to return to a life of dialysis and await a second organ. With developing medical technology, the variety of possible donors—including brain-dead, heart-dead, and living—has greatly increased. Nevertheless, the body can reject others' organs, even with increasingly successful immunosuppressants, so once a recipient has tried an organ transplant, they may have to continue to receive organs until their end of lives.

ATTITUDES TO ORGAN RECEPTION

Organ reception is a vital lifeline and the most important event for concerned parties to organ transplantation. Most all recipients are very happy to receive organs, but attitudes to organ reception are very varied and complex, reflecting not only individual values and family interactions but also social ethics and national and broader cultural responses.

1. Needs of Recipients before Transplantation

The fundamental principle of organ transplantation is that of the "gift of life": it depends on organs that become available because of the altruism of donors. Most recipients, on the other hand, are only able to consider their own needs because they are critically ill. Organ transplant candidates are preparing for their own deaths and cannot give much thought to the donor's death and the donor family's grief: they just hope for successful medical treatment of their illness.

2. Reactions of the Recipient's Family

Family attitudes to organ reception differ with different organs. For a heart transplant, for example, organ donation is only possible from a brain-dead donor so the recipient's family must meet high financial costs, sometimes gathering money by asking passers-by on the street for donations to enable them to go and take care of the patient in a foreign country. With a kidney donation it may be possible to receive an organ from a living donor, so the recipient's family must consider becoming donors themselves because of the current severe organ shortage. The most serious problem then is who will donate the organ to the family recipient, taking into account both their own medical condition and the problems that may arise from emotional family ties. Organ reception places a heavy burden on the recipient's family members.

3. Opinions of Individual Family Members

Every member of a recipient's family will have different opinions about organ reception, reflected in their own status within the family and their individual feelings, which may vary depending on whether the donor is brain-dead or living. Recipients of hearts from brain-dead donors usually expect to become donors on their deaths, but their parents do not always agree to donate their recipient children's organs, sometimes refusing to allow specific organs or even any organs to be donated. When patients receive kidneys from living donors (who are only allowed to be family members in Japan) the relationship between recipient and donor is an important element and the opinions of family members can vary widely, especially when the recipient's health may fluctuate after the operation.

4. Advocacy of Medical Professionals

An organ transplant medical professional's mission is successful organ transplantation from a donor, with a safe and fair operation from harvest to transplant. In reality, however, there are few domestic brain-dead donors and most recipients depend on living and overseas donors, regardless of global ethical and sometimes legal problems. While medical staff advocate organ transplantation, their opinions vary over the issues of living donors and overseas transplants, although most develop their own philosophy based on actual practical conditions. Nevertheless, they have to weigh up the importance of the recipient's and the donor's lives, regardless of the donor's status.

5. Attitudes of Recipients after Transplantation

Attitudes of successful organ recipients are varied and ambivalent: all feel gratitude, but this can work on their lives in a very positive or unthinkably negative way. Some work to promote organ donation, while some struggle with ways to repay the donor or donor's family for their organ, but an impression of recipients being too happy and enjoying their life can be hard for donor families to take during their grieving process. A few feel guilty for receiving an organ before others who were on the waiting list with them for years. Others feel overwhelmed because the gift they have been given is so great.

6. Recipients' Assessments of Donors

Recipients' assessments of their donors are often connected with the organs involved.

1. Hearts can only be received from brain-dead donors, and heart recipients' assessments of the donations are of wonderful human altruism. Some recipients, especially child recipients, believe that the donor family must feel happy to donate an organ for others to live.
2. Livers can be received from brain-dead and living donors (as partial liver donations). Most liver donations worldwide come from brain-dead donors, but in Japan they are mostly from living donors. While heart donation involves one donor and one recipient,

liver donation has more alternatives: usually one liver is transplanted into plural recipients as a partial liver transplant, a split liver transplant, or a "domino" transplant (transplanting the original recipient's liver into another patient). Since living liver donation is possible, recipients sometimes expect living donations from their family circle but a family donor candidate can often be hesitant, as liver transplantation is a very invasive and complex procedure.

3. Liver recipients often want to donate their own organs to someone in return, but the liver transplant process can be very high risk, so becoming a living donor is very dangerous. Transplant surgeons expect cadaveric donors, including both brain-dead and heart-dead donors, because of the high risks to living donors. Most Japanese recipients have to go abroad to receive an organ from a foreign donor and this creates additional difficult emotions and assessments of donors. Most Japanese liver recipients went to Australia; the reason for this is not clear but Australian hospitals are now banned from accepting Japanese recipients since the Istanbul Declaration.

4. Kidney recipients will be on a waiting list for an average of fourteen years or more, awaiting a donation from a brain-dead or heart-dead donor or a living donor from either the family circle or another south Asian country; they mostly view organ donation as a valuable gift from the donor.

5. Many kidney recipients rely on someone from within their family circle—including parents, children, siblings, and spouses—under Japanese organ transplantation law. They are therefore somewhat ambivalent about the donation and both hesitate and feel guilt over their family member's sacrifice.

6. Recently, retransplant surgery has become more viable and popular, and recipients may have multiple donors. They tend to be more sensitive to the donor of the most recently transplanted organ in the recipient's body than former donors. However, the combinations of donors can vary from patient to patient so more research is needed in this area.

7. Recipients' Families' Assessments of Donors

1. It does not make much difference to recipients' families whether a donor is brain-dead or heart-dead, but they do care about receiving organs within their family circle. Some say that cadaveric organ transplantation "shames the family," so organ reception is a matter not only for an individual recipient but also for their family in Japan. This way of thinking reflects Japanese traditional belief and the historical background that still remains in the heart of Japanese

notions about organ donation/reception, which evokes Japanese "shame culture," which places emphasis on public opinion (as opposed to the Western "guilt culture," which places emphasis on religious teaching) (Benedict 1946).

2. Living donors are not seen as shaming a family, but the problem arises with who may donate to whom within family circles. For example, a recipient candidate tries to arrange organ transplantation from a living donor within his family. Relatives on his mother's side expect his father to donate and vice versa. If the organ transplant surgery is successful all remains peaceful, but if the operation fails, or if either or both parties suffer poor health after surgery, family members' relationships can become difficult.

3. Many Japanese recipients depend on overseas donations from brain-dead donors, meaning that the family has to gather money from charitable donations for the recipient to go overseas.[1] According to my data, one recipient father was against begging for money on the street: he developed his own business and made the money that way because he felt that he had no guarantee of taking his daughter alive back to Japan to say thank you to the people who donated money. In Japanese culture, people are likely to feel comfortable and give money easily with sympathy for a very sick child, but the father assumes an obligation to the person who gave his daughter money. "Obligation" is at the core of Japanese culture: once a Japanese person feels under an obligation, the need to repay is incredibly strong.

4. Most Japanese liver recipients depend on living partial liver donors, but this operation is more invasive than the equivalent for living kidney donors and has high levels of risk for the donor. Some recipients (mostly mothers) want to donate even though they might die as a result of the operation; some family recipients are concerned about the attendant risks but feel they can't say no because it is expected of them; some do say no and cause rifts within the family, either because of the risks or because they are against the idea of organ donation in principle. This can cause extensive problems within family groups.

5. Numbers of retransplant operations have been increasing and recipients may have multiple donors from inside the traditional and expanding legal family circle, which may include further removed relatives. The relationships between a recipient and donors in the family are unpredictable; this is a high-priority new area of research.

The next section introduces recipients' narratives, paying particular attention to the status of the donor.

RECIPIENTS' NARRATIVES

The attitudes of recipients to the time spent waiting for an organ and their reactions on receipt vary dramatically. They develop their own unique philosophy and try to put an individual rational interpretation on the process. All recipients also have great appreciation for donors and their organs, but have different depths of gratitude toward donor families; not all recognize the donor family's involvement and the issues that may surround their decision to donate their loved one's organ. The recipients' gratitude is immensely—sometimes overwhelmingly—strong, and many struggle with ways to try to reciprocate for the organ donation. In general, a recipient's gratitude is much stronger toward an unknown brain-dead donor than toward a living family member donor.

Unsurprisingly, recipients responded very differently to interview questions about their own processes of organ reception, depending on the different organ received and the different donor type (brain-dead, heart-dead, or living). Some gave very brief answers, partly owing to their physical infirmity, some whispered hesitantly and apologetically, while others answered proudly. But even when appearing to be cheery and light-hearted, many gave anxious glances every now and then, and some of their comments showed that they had given profound consideration to their life and its meaning. When touching on the topic of donors and their families, all recipients looked grim and became quiet. It became clear that recipients do not know how to appreciate donors fully or how to contact and behave toward a donor family.

Recipients' Gratitude

All recipients are immensely grateful for the organ transplant that enabled them to survive, but while setting a very high value on it, they draw different meanings and inferences from the term "organ transplantation." It is wrong to believe that all recipients have the same appreciation for organ transplantation with a single simple view, as their assessments and ways of offering appreciation are very diverse and complex. Sometimes their appreciation encourages them to live their life fully and in a particular manner, but sometimes their appreciation feels too strong to bear and they feel it as a burdensome weight.

In Japanese society it is customary to exchange gifts twice a year in "Oseibo" (December) and "Ochugen" (June), and the duty of reciprocation is felt very strongly by both gift senders and receivers as a social function and traditional custom. This tradition affects the Japanese concept of gift giving and receiving, and is associated with the low number of organ donations in Japan, which has caused the most severe organ shortage in the world (Lock 2002). Because recipients feel uncomfortable accepting a gift that is not material and thus not possible to return in kind or with an equivalent sum of money, the social gift-giving function is impaired and the inability of recipients to reciprocate leads to emotional guilt. As a result, most recipients try to produce a unique present or idea to give in return.

Recipient Satoshi's Organ Reception — "The Most Precious Gift in the World"

Recipient Satoshi is thirty-five years old, single, university educated, and a company employee, living with his parents. He received a simultaneous pancreas and kidney transplant from a brain-dead donor at the age of thirty-three in Japan.

> I really appreciate it. I can't express how grateful I am. . . . It was a really cold day and it looked like snow; when I came back from dialysis and turned on a heater, the phone rang and they said, "We have a donor!" The suddenness of it caught me by surprise, yes: the news of a donor was too sudden to absorb without any advance notice. I don't remember anything about the organ transplant. I was lying in bed when I regained consciousness and the surgery was over. . . . I'm grateful to be alive now, because I was too severely ill to survive without an organ transplant at that time. Without the transplant I would not exist any longer and I would have died already. . . . I don't have to be overcome with terror of a hypoglycemic attack anymore; also, after so many years without being able to create urine, I just wanted to urinate by myself and actually I had been dreaming of wetting my bed! . . . Organ transplantation is the most precious gift and behavior in this world. All I can do is. . . . I always live in thankfulness and try take care of my health to live with the received organs as long as possible. I can't thank the donor, donor family and my doctors enough.

This recipient's was the third simultaneous pancreas and kidney transplant from a brain-dead donor in Japan and his narrative is very rare and valuable. It reveals the process of receiving an organ transplant from brain-dead donors, highlighting the speed required to complete the operation, which allows the recipient no time to contemplate or absorb the news beforehand. He is grateful not only to his donor, the donor family, and medical staff but also to his family members, developing medical technology, the organ transplantation law, and his own luck for his chance of survival. His quality of life improved considerably and he felt free of the fear of dying from both hypoglycemia and being anuric (unable to create urine).

1. Satoshi's motivations for organ reception were twofold: he was so critically ill that he was unlikely to live much longer without the transplant, and he also wanted to come off dialysis and be able to urinate by himself, and to be free from fear of hypoglycemia. One of the most valuable physiological phenomena perceived by kidney organ recipient candidates is to make their own urine. This fact

is usually unknown to the donor family. As a result, receiving thanks from a recipient for being able to make urine as a result of a donated organ can generate opposition and ill-will between recipients and donor families because of a lack of understanding of the issues.

2. His organ transplant surgery was performed only a few years after the Japanese organ transplantation law was established, so he had no chance to learn about the operation in advance from experienced recipients. As an early organ recipient he faced this unknown operation with a mixture of hope and anxiety for both himself (and his family members) and the transplant surgeons. As a result, he developed strong ties with the surgeons and his appreciation for others after the operation was much wider than some recipients.

3. In spite of their pride in the country's advanced medical technology, many Japanese are very conservative and organ transplantation is still taboo in many parts of Japan. As a result, Satoshi only told his parents about his surgery, feeling the need to hide it from all other family and neighbors, for fear of being accused of shameful behavior, or even cannibalism.

4. This is the only narrative data from a simultaneous pancreas and kidney transplant recipient so far. In addition, Satoshi's donor was a Japanese brain-dead donor, of which there have still been very few, so future research may need to focus on gaining information from other similar recipients to enable comparison of narratives.

Recipient Ai's Organ Reception — "I Fear of Death Overseas"

Recipient Ai is thirty years old, single, high-school educated, and unemployed, living with her father, mother, and an older sister. She received a liver transplant from a brain-dead donor at the age of twenty-two in Australia.

> I faced a daily life-or-death struggle. I felt that my body had gradually become not my own. My way of life became no way to live: I lost control of my body. I was reduced to a skeleton, just skin and bones, and only my belly was bulging like pregnant lady with massive ascites of about 3 kg, almost the same as a baby's weight. . . . I couldn't even hold chopsticks to eat rice, walk on my own legs, or roll over in bed: trying to move my body a little to the right or left in bed used up all my energy. . . . Because I was incredibly ill, I contemplated whether I should try to live without a reason to live, and had great inner conflict. I couldn't sleep in Australia despite being very tired because I was so scared that once I fell asleep I might never wake up. I was reeling with such fear every day and night, and spent many sleepless nights worrying about my own death . . . it was just too painful for me!

Recipient Hana's Organ Reception — "I Feel Survivor's Guilt"

Recipient Hana is twenty-three years old, married, high-school educated, and a part-time employee, living with her husband (who is also a kidney recipient). She received a liver transplant from a brain-dead donor at the age of fourteen in Australia.

> What could I do when I was only thirteen years old? Could I refuse? For me, the overseas transplant was portrayed as a short-stay English program for high-school students. In Japan, the doctors and my parents decided all my medical treatment plans, so I flew to Australia just obeying their wishes. However, when I arrived in the Australian hospital, a nurse asked me, "Do you really want to be a recipient? Do you really want to live with a donated organ?" How could I answer? Could I say no? . . . In Australia, they require an organ reception will even from children. My room had eight Japanese liver candidate children and everyone was waiting for a liver from an Australian brain-dead donor. These eight candidates' conditions varied from mild to serious and we could see the patients in the most serious condition and those who were not so critical. I was only mildly symptomatic at that time. All the Japanese candidate children awaiting organs in the Australian hospital dreamed of being healthy ladies. Although my symptoms were the mildest I received the organ because I had the highest possibility of survival. My more seriously ill Japanese friends either suffered organ rejection or did not have a chance to receive an organ: I was the only child in that room who survived. . . . That waiting room felt like a game of Russian roulette. I blame myself for receiving the organ: if one of the other girls had received the liver she might have been a more suitable recipient. If everybody had survived, I would be happy but that is impossible, so I don't want to think about my organ reception . . . the memory is too hard for me, too tough!

These two liver recipients' narratives describe the difficult conditions of overseas transplants: the first struggled with her physical symptoms and fear of death in a foreign country but the second suffered mental pressure from receiving an organ: she felt guilty to be the only successful recipient in a waiting room of Japanese children in a foreign hospital. While these recipients did not regret the overseas transplant, both suffered greatly as a result—one before and one after organ reception— because by hoping for an organ donation they felt they were waiting for someone's death, although in reality they were simply waiting for an organ to be donated, not hoping that someone would die.

1. Ai was informed by her doctor of the need for an overseas transplant to survive and she consented eventually, while Hana was still a child (under fifteen years old), so her parents consented on her behalf: she just obeyed her doctors' and parents' decision about the overseas transplant. She flew to an Australian hospital, where the attitude to children's rights is different from that in Japan, and

children have more of a voice in their medical decisions. The nurse asked her, "Are you sure you want this organ transplant?" but from her cultural background and the language barrier she felt that she had no choice but to say "Yes."

2. When Ai was first informed about overseas organ transplantation by her doctor she was tempted but could not say yes immediately as she could not meet the 2 million USD cost at that time. Her mother asked her true feelings toward the operation, setting aside financial considerations. When she replied, "Who wants to die?" all her family members made all kinds of plans to support her and started to raise money to help her.

3. Hana was still a child and her family reached consensus on how to proceed without her input. (Usually Japanese parents reach consent with children's doctors and the children have no opportunity to take part in the decision-making process themselves.) She flew to Australia as if she was going on school exchange program, but once she arrived she was asked to declare her organ reception will so she had to decide and answer in her own words.

Recipient Hiroshi's Organ Reception — "I Was Waiting for Someone's Death"

Recipient Hiroshi is sixty years old, married, university educated, and an association administrator, living with his wife. He received a kidney transplant from a brain-dead donor at the age of forty-three in the United States.

> Although there are many expressions to describe organ donation, including the "gift of life," "gift of love," or "relay of life," I think now that it is really a "given life." Yes, I think that I was given life from the bottom of my heart. I'm alive now: this means that I was reborn from my almost dead body. I couldn't have survived without a donor; I can't live without a donor's organ now. My life's existence has been supported not only by the donor but also by medical staff, family members, and friends. When I received an organ I thought immediately that "God is always on my mind." Having this idea, I will be able to be forgiven by the donor and donor family, and I want them to understand my feelings. . . . Organ transplantation is not a normal medical treatment, because I had to wait for a person's death and for them to donate an organ to me: this is really hard to go through as a medical treatment. . . . Organ transplantation is a medical treatment that requires mental toughness from recipients; it is not a simple treatment. Recipients have two kinds of pain: physical pain from kidney failure and the psychological pain of waiting for someone's death. Antagonistic feelings seemed to go round and round in my head: recipients have to swing between two feelings of "I want to live with someone's organ" and "I have to wait for someone's death." I'm selfish, aren't I? I suffered kidney failure and I couldn't take dialysis so I had to wait to die

on a waiting list in a Japanese hospital. Because I have no siblings and my parents had passed away, I couldn't depend on a living donor, but I had to battle with my selfish need for survival! I wanted to get better but my dreams told me I needed to go to the United States and wait for someone's death and receive an American donor's kidney to survive. I knew this was false and that I had at least a few years ahead of me without organ reception in the U.S. hospital. But I was aware that many donors had passed away already, so I was holding out for a donor's precious organ as long as I could to show my appreciation and beg his forgiveness! Once we become recipients we have to hold on to the heavy-hearted feeling of guilt over the donor's death forever.

Recipient Ken's Organ Reception—"I Was Preparing for Death"

Recipient Ken is sixty-two years old, married, university educated, and retired, living with his wife, oldest daughter, and second daughter. He received a kidney transplant from a brain-dead donor at the age of fifty-seven in the United States.

In my case, I had a more difficult time than others because I was ineligible for dialysis. So I would like to inform to people all over the world how wonderful organ transplantation is! Many people don't know that Japan is the most underdeveloped country for organ transplantation. . . . I'd like show that I am back on my feet! I want to live as long as possible to tell everyone about this unbelievable medical technology. I got angry and took my anger out on my wife; then I became depressed and was preparing for my death because I had kidney failure but dialysis did not help me. My fellow patients who were on dialysis died one after the other, and I thought that it was my turn next. . . . Fortunately, my friend (Hiroshi) wrote a letter to an American transplant surgeon and I survived. . . . I have become so healthy and so happy now and treat my family better but I also want to volunteer to help as many people as possible to become successful organ recipients. I haven't written a thank you letter yet. Because my donor was an American car accident victim, I wonder whether his family members wanted to save an American recipient not a Japanese one. I suspect if they knew I was Japanese they might feel disappointment and regret at their organ donation decision. However, I should say thank you to them. That's my only matter of concern now. I decided that after five years I will be able to complete a marathon, and then I will be able to write a thank you letter to the donor family in the United States. I can't write in English but I will write a Japanese letter and ask my friend to translate it. It will be a great excuse to write to them: I became healthy enough to complete the Tokyo marathon with your donated organ! This evidence is very objective so maybe the donor family will be able to understand how much my health condition has improved to enable me to run and how much I appreciate their organ donation decision and their family member's donated organ.

These two overseas transplant recipients, who received organs from brain-dead donors, are friends. Hiroshi introduced his doctor in the United States to Ken, who depended on Hiroshi not only for medical advice but also for an English translation of his thank you letter and for communicating with other American recipients at international organ transplant events. Both are very grateful to the brain-dead donors, although Hiroshi has very complex feelings about the donation. One of the main reasons for his overseas transplant was that he had no living family donors in the 1980s, but he worked in the United States for some years and an American friend told him about American transplant surgery in Ohio. He took the chance and flew to Ohio, where he was the only Japanese kidney patient in the heart transplant section. Heart donors often appeared but not kidney donors, so he waited for a long time, during which his thoughts turned from waiting for a kidney to waiting for a kidney donation, then for a kidney donor, then a deceased donor, then waiting for someone's death. Some recipients recognize that organ donation cannot happen without someone's death so they blame themselves for waiting for a donation which must result from that death. He said that he felt so selfish and was now begging forgiveness from the donor and donor family through his prayers every night.

Recipient Akira's Organ Reception — "I Want to Show My Appreciation"

Recipient Akira is fifty-five years old, married, high-school educated, and a company employee, living with his mother, wife, oldest daughter, and second daughter. He received a kidney transplant from a brain-dead donor at the age of forty in Japan.

> Of course, I really appreciate the donor and donor family donating the organ: now I can survive and I have lived without dialysis for fifteen years. However, I can't thank the donor and donor family, as they are entitled to anonymity under the present organ transplantation law so I don't know who they are. This makes it difficult for us recipients to show our appreciation for their donation. There is no point of contact, although organ transplantation creates a sort of touchstone between donor and recipient for the first time. Recipients feel gratitude toward the donor and donor family after organ reception. But before the surgery I neither expected nor hoped for someone's death at all. In fact, while someone died and donated an organ, someone suffered kidney failure and needed an organ transplant separately, and only the organ transplant surgery connected the donor and recipient. So the recipient feels gratitude to the donor and donor family and this grows daily. However, the donor passed away, so only we can say thank you to their bereaved family, which creates a new relationship between donor family and recipient. . . . Some deceased people donate their organs to us recipients, and we thank the donor and donor family and create imaginary relationships with the deceased donor and real relationships

with donor families through transplant events, etc. That's my own phi-losophy about organ transplantation. . . . But my philosophy has changed since organ reception. My physical quality of life has become unpredictably better and my feelings of gratitude have also grown. And I'm troubled about how I can show my appreciation to the donor and donor family. This is something I wonder about and grapple with every day.

Recipient Takeshi's Organ Reception — "I Received a Second Organ"

Recipient Takeshi is thirty-two years old, single, high-school educat-ed, and unemployed, living with his grandparents, mother, and younger brother. He received two kidney transplants: the first from a living donor (his mother) at the age of fourteen and the second from a heart-dead donor at the age of twenty-five in Japan.

> I thank both the donor who donated an organ and the donor family who gave informed consented about organ donation. . . . In Japan we can't receive a kidney easily even when we are on a waiting list. Kid-ney recipient candidates say things like "Few people are able to receive an organ," "There is trouble getting a donated organ," "We have been be eagerly waiting for the opportunity to receive an organ for more than ten years but we haven't," and "You know, organ transplantation can't be done without a donor!" Although I'm glad to have received a new organ twice, I'm really sorry for my mother the living donor, and I really appreciate the second unknown heart-dead donor. I'm very blessed because the second organ has given me a second chance, and some patients never even receive one kidney. Of course, the first and the second transplant were different—I mean my feelings were differ-ent: I was vividly aware of the second organ! The difference in enthu-siasm for the organ reception was clear: I strongly felt that this was the second organ for me, and I should have a high regard for it. Regardless of being unconscious of it, I regret my first organ donation from my mother and I feel very sorry, even though I was a child and knew nothing about it. The first organ reception and the second are absolute-ly different for me. . . . To be honest, there was no choice for me—I know that some patients have a hesitation but in my case, I just thought about organ transplantation. When I needed dialysis as a child, my mother started examinations to donate her kidney for me, so the first organ, the dialysis, and the second organ are just a sequence of treat-ment for me. Since I have depended on organ transplantation, I ac-knowledge the importance of organ donors, but I don't know how they feel and what they think about recipients.

These four kidney recipients' narratives describe how difficult it is for patients to live on dialysis and how much they eagerly await the oppor-tunity to have an organ transplant to be free from it. While they all re-ceived kidneys, three of them were donated from brain-dead donors (one in Japan and two in Ohio, in the United States).

1. Hiroshi had an overseas transplant in 1985 when it was not yet common, but he had a cosmopolitan job and was comfortable flying to an American hospital. He survived and lives in Japan, where he introduced the American hospital to his fellow patients and gradually it became known all over the world. He was one of the first overseas transplant recipients, but this is now a popular option for organ donation candidates, causing a worldwide problem that has given rise to the WHO principles calling for member countries to discourage people from going abroad for transplant surgery.

2. While it is clear that an organ donation is required for a transplant, some recipients accept this fact as a feature of the treatment, but others assesses that organ transplantation is a process of "waiting for someone's death." Hiroshi felt this way in hospital in the United States, and he advised other recipient candidates to develop a toughness of their character. He insists that recipients are special because they experienced a miraculous return to life and can only share this special experience with each other. Ken did not mention negative feelings toward organ transplantation, but was wondering how he was going to write a thank you letter to his donor family in the United States. Akira had come to terms with his feelings about organ reception but was struggling to find a way to repay the donor and the donor family one day.

3. Akira had no contact with the donor before the organ transplant, but afterwards he felt as if he had the donor's and even the donor family's kindness inside his body, and he created an imaginary relationship with the donor and an internalized relationship with the surviving donor's family. He is a member of an organ transplant recipients association and he tries to keep in contact with the organ donors association to forge a relationship with donor families. The association has attended many events; at some of them, such as the international and national "Transplant Games" (similar to the Paralympics), recipients and medical staff invite donor families as guests.

4. As medical technology develops, retransplantation is increasing and recipients may have multiple donors of different statuses, including living, heart-dead, and brain-dead. Takeshi's attitude is very complicated and changed between his first and second organ receptions. Because he was a child at the time of the first donation from his (living) mother, he was too young to understand organ transplantation and consent was only required from his parents and the doctors. As noted earlier, recipient candidates who are children are kept uninformed and do not have an opportunity to announce their organ reception wills. Takeshi's first organ failed after just one year, after which he was waiting for a second kidney

for ten years. In Japan, even kidney recipients face a severe organ shortage so they have to be on the waiting list frequently more than ten years (an average of fourteen years). During this time he changed his assessment of organ donation and donors. His second organ transplantation from an unknown heart-dead donor made him feel twice as happy and grateful, both for this second organ and for his mother's original organ donation.

5. These different attitudes to organ reception are also connected to the varied experiences of each recipient's progress from dialysis to organ transplantation, and to the kind of donor, whether brain-dead, heart-dead, or living, and whether domestic or overseas. In addition, the duration of the wait for organs is also an important factor: the longer the waiting time, the more likely the recipient is to confuse waiting for an organ with waiting for someone's death, which can cause feelings of deep guilt. Some people in Japan regard organ transplantation as an unbearable treatment involving waiting for someone's death, and are against both organ donation and reception. Many Japanese recipients feel happiness for their improved physical condition but guilt from the psychological weight on their minds.

It is difficult to generalize about recipients' reactions because each has a different history before successful organ reception, with a variety of different experiences leading to the operation. According to the narrative data, organ transplantation leads to some very dramatic stories and narratives are changing daily following the development of this emerging medical technology. All recipients feel some ambivalence about the organ transplantation process. Satoshi feels great gratitude toward his donor but still hides his organ reception from everyone except his parents. Ai thanks her donor for her donated liver and has constructed a subservient relationship, deciding to become a donor of tissue, bone, and corneas herself at the end of her life in a reciprocal act. Hana is grateful to her donor but feels that the gift of a liver is too heavy a responsibility, both as a result of her guilt at the other patient's deaths, and because she feels she must strive to be healthy even when feeling sick or depressed because she has someone else's organ to look after. Hiroshi actively advocates overseas transplantation, but begs for both appreciation and forgiveness in his prayers every night. Ken recommends organ transplantation for a transplant organization but he cannot write a thank you letter yet as he hopes to spare the donor family's feelings. Akira thinks of organ donation and reception as separate, but since receiving a donated organ has been trying to find a way to show his gratitude to the donor and donor family. Takeshi recognizes that organ transplantation is part of his therapy, but he feels sorry for the first donor (his mother) and has twice as great an appreciation for both organs since his second organ reception.

"Transplanted Life"

"Transplanted life" is a term coined by a transplant physician in Japan who accepts Japanese patients with serious heart failure who will die without a heart transplant. Because there are so few Japanese heart donors, he sends or accompanies his transplant candidates to a U.S. hospital. According to him, recipients should forget their "first" lives from birth to organ transplantation and should consider their "rebirth" after organ reception as a second life: so-called "transplanted life." Many recipients imagine the "gift of life" that organ donation will offer them through rose-tinted spectacles, but organ transplantation is not magic. Although the recipient can be liberated from the conditions of organ failure they are suffering, organ transplants do not combat the health threat posed by rejection and recipients have to take immunosuppressant drugs for the rest of their lives.

"Transplanted life" has both uniformities and ambivalences for recipients, in a similar way that transplant surgeons and recipient and donor coordinators have varied feelings about organ transplantation as medical professionals. All recipients are grateful to donors (and donor families), but their assessments of organ transplantation itself are difficult to evaluate and may include strong feelings of guilt for the donors, their bereaved families, and other unsuccessful organ reception candidates they have outlived. Organ donation and reception are very sensitive issues, affected by individuals' life values, social consensus, and other factors. Some recipients are proud of their organ reception but some hide the secret from relatives, neighbors, and the public. "Transplanted life"[2] is not easy in Japan, where organ recipients' lives are still veiled in secrecy.

All recipients struggle to accept their donor's "gift of life" in their own way. They often feel that they cannot offer enough thanks for such a priceless precious gift and wonder (and ask donors) what they can do in return. If an "okaeshi" (token of appreciation) is too precious, valuable, and rare, the recipient becomes beholden to the donor. While grateful for these organ donations, the recipients want to repay donors to the best of their ability but do not know how: they cannot give back an organ or an equivalent sum of money to the donors and donor families. This unreturnable gift causes great difficulties in Japanese society, which has strong ties to traditional culture and mores, even in the most modern situations such as those surrounding emerging medical technologies. Marcel Mauss's description of the "norm of reciprocity" is a helpful guide to assist anthropologists in understanding the feelings of recipients and the essential problems of organ transplantation (Mauss 1954). Fox and Swazey also focus on the fundamental problems of organ donation and reception and organ replacement treatment in their book on "spare parts" (Fox and Swazey 1992).

NOTES

1. Most child recipients have to rely on overseas transplants, but this costs billions of yen (millions of U.S. dollars) so the recipient's family members have to beg for charitable donations. During my fieldwork, I saw a picture labeled "Save my brother!" in which two little girls were trying to raise money outside a public place for their elder brother's overseas heart transplant.

2. During my research I interviewed several organ recipients and learned of their experiences. Meg was a young liver recipient who had an overseas transplant. Her boyfriend was the fortunate recipient of two kidney donations: the first from a living donor and the second from a heart-dead donor. Furthermore, he was the dependent of a middle-aged man who was also a kidney recipient (from a brain-dead donor). We all had a tofu (soy bean curd) dinner together because Meg can't eat meat or raw fish. The three recipients seemed like father, brother, and sister. Meg took a photograph of the three of us for me, and whenever I look at this picture, I realize that if we had banned organ transplantation, the image would never have existed and all three recipients would have passed away more than fifteen or twenty years ago.

REFERENCES

Benedict, R. (1946). *The Chrysanthemum and the Sword: Patterns of Japanese Culture*. Boston, MA: Houghton Mifflin.

Fox, R., and Swazey, J. (1992). *Spare Parts: Organ Replacement in American Society*. New York: Oxford University Press.

Inhorn, M., and Wentzell, E. (2011). "Embodying Emergent Masculinities: Reproductive and Sexual Health Technologies in the Middle East and Mexico." *American Ethnologist* 38(4), 801–815.

Lock, M. (2002). *Twice Dead: Organ Transplants and the Reinvention of Death*. Berkeley: University of California Press.

Mauss, M. (1954). *The Gift: Forms and Functions of Exchange in Archaic Societies*, translated by I. Cunnison. London: Cohen and West Ltd.

Yasuoka, M. K. (2006). "Rebirthable Life: Medical Anthropology Study of the Concept of Life According to Concerned Parties Involved in Brain Death and Organ Transplantation." PhD thesis: Department of History and Anthropology (Medical Anthropology), Graduate School of Letters, Hokkaido University, Sapporo, Japan (unpublished).

———. (2010). "Medical Refugees in Japan: From Overseas Transplants to Organ Self-Sufficiency for Japanese Recipients." *Applied Ethics: Challenges for the 21st Century*. Sapporo, Japan: Center for Applied Ethics and Philosophy, Hokkaido University, 85–97.

FOUR

Narratives of Donor Families

INTRODUCTION

There was no room to think about organ reception when I saw cheerful recipients, especially when I participated in the transplant games. . . . When I watched their happy figures, to be honest, I thought that they would be more, what should I say, more sick. . . . Though I didn't think recipients used wheelchairs, but I thought that they would play sports slowly and with more difficulty: I was surprised at that time, the recipients were such strong players. But on the other hand, well, I thought at that time, "Why are you recipients so cheerful?" On the contrary, what should I say my feeling at that time. I know, it's a little difficult to make people understand, also it's too difficult to say to someone by myself, though, I thought "Why are you, recipients so fine? Can you pretend more sick persons?" To be honest, I have such a feeling at that time. Honestly speaking, my head knows that but. . . . Of course I understand the feeling that it is wonderful for them, recipients to be a much better health condition though. . . . My most honest feelings is why are there my daughter in there with cheerful people. That's my honest and true feelings! — A donor father's narrative

Organ donation is an essential element in conducting organ transplant surgery and offering recipients the "gift of life" based on altruism from donors' organ donation wills and donor families' agreement to honor them. There is, however, no way to learn the feelings of the deceased organ donors directly, so we have to rely on the narratives of their families as those closest to them and most directly affected. This chapter introduces a number of narratives from organ donors' family members to understand both the donors' wills and the variety of donor families' decision-making processes.

All parties recognize the necessity of organ donations for transplantation, but while transplant surgeons and recipients await a donation with anticipation, for donor family members the decision to allow an organ to be harvested is one of the toughest and cruelest procedures they will have to face. The donor family plays a crucial role in the decision-making process for organ donation and reactions to the situation vary widely. The narratives that follow are categorized by family relationship with the donor (father/child, mother/child, and wife/husband), giving an indication of the variety of different perspectives and emotions involved, as well as the motivations behind the decision.

Tracing the diversity of donor families' struggles after the decision to make a donation is also important in order to understand the dark side of organ transplantation treatment. As seen through their narratives, the emotions they battle with—from grief to sublimation of the donor's death and regret at the organ donation decision—should not be ignored. Not only in Japan but also in other countries, people and mass communication media tend to look only at recipients, even though transplantation could not take place without organ donations. Yet the sudden and dramatic experiences of donor families are a useful textbook that can help others to understand the unique background of the world of Japanese organ transplantation. Unfortunately, these narratives are extremely rare for three reasons:

1. Organ transplantation is a cutting-edge medical technology that has only recently given rise to the relatively new category of the donor as a medical agent who can control concerned parties such as recipients, donor families, and transplant surgeons.
2. In order to protect the privacy of donor families, it is difficult to contact them and very unusual to receive permission to record their narratives via interview.
3. Although the first Japanese heart transplant operation took place in 1968 and the first organ transplantation law was established in Japan in 1997, no transplants were performed between 1969 and 1998, so the Japanese organ shortage problem is the most severe worldwide, meaning that Japanese donor families' narratives are very rare data (Yasuoka 2004 and 2006).

ORGAN DONATION FOR DONOR FAMILIES

Organ donation produces a variety of ambivalent feelings in all parties. For transplant surgeons, organ donation is a significant medical contribution enabling them to save a recipient following a patient's death. Conversely, they may feel guilty because they were not able to save the donor's life. In addition, during the same procedure, surgeons have the temporary illusion of killing the donor with their own hands by harvesting a beating heart, even though the donor is brain-dead and has little or no chance of returning to life. Recipients are grateful for the altruism of donors, which enables them to receive organs and thus delivers the chance of survival through this "gift of life." Nevertheless, they are also aware that by hoping to receive an organ they are anticipating another person's death, which gives rise to very mixed emotions.

Donor families also face a mixture of feelings as they assess a doctor's offer to harvest their family member's organs to try to save another patient. Organ donation turns a bereaved family into a donor family (one interviewee scolded me, saying: "I'm not a bereaved parent! Call me a donor parent because my son is alive inside someone's body, even [if it's] only his organ!"). How do donor families come to terms with the idea of donating the organs of a beloved family member? How do they negotiate between their altruistic decision to allow organs to be used to save a life and the resistance in their heart of hearts toward agreeing to let a surgeon harvest their loved one's organs? Most donor families are on a roller-coaster of emotions and swing between personal sadness and rational judgment in a very short time, since the decision to harvest an organ must frequently be made rapidly.

The donor families' narratives show that three important factors have great influence over their decision to donate an organ—the motivation for the donation, the way the family's decision-making process is handled, and their sentiments toward the idea of organ donation and its results. When a donor has an organ donation will or donor card, this becomes the strongest motivation for organ donation as it allows the family to rest assured that the donor wanted his or her organs to be used. In the absence of such a will, the family members have to rely on their own feelings about organ donation and about what the donor might have wanted. In addition, when donor family members can discuss and decide freely among themselves the after-effects are easier to deal with; however, when a family feels that medical staff have forced them into organ donation or family members suffer mental abuse over the decision from their relatives and neighbors, they grieve longer and much more deeply. The decision is also affected by the family members' attitudes to the idea of organ donation, which may range from regret over an organ being removed from their loved one's body to satisfaction at a donation will being fulfilled, or a combination of both, as well as other emotions. Careful attention to the donor families' narratives sheds fascinating light on the diversity, complexity, and sensitivity of all these factors in the organ donation decision-making process.

MOTIVATION

Several different motives may lie behind a family's decision to proceed with organ donation.

1. Existence of a Donation Will

The ideal case occurs when a donor has made a donation will in writing and informed his or her family members of its existence, especially when all family members know about the will and all agree that organ donation is the right action. In this case the donation not only stands as the donor's testament but also fuels the donor family's mission to respond to the deceased's wishes: organ donation can help to heal the donor family's grief as they fulfill the donor's wishes, rather than causing rifts and differing opinions.

2. Presumption of a Donation Will

In some cases it is not clear whether an organ donation will has been written, but all family members know that the donor was in favor of organ donation as a result of a direct discussion or a preference made clear by behavior. In these circumstances it is relatively easy for the donor family to presume that a donation will was intended to make a smooth decision on organ donation.

3. Doctor's Recommendation

After the original organ transplantation law was established in Japan in 1997, the most common motivation for a bereaved family to donate organs was a medical professional's recommendation. Most donor families did not consider organ donation issues until a beloved family member became brain-dead. At this stage, a transplant surgeon could take the opportunity to recommend organ donation to a bereaved family, who might be overcome by a family member's sudden death. This can be perceived as an ideal opportunity for both transplant surgeons and recipients, but they are in different situations from the donor family, and it is a myth that donor families are always happy to donate organs to save recipients, regardless of their internal dilemmas.

4. Pressure from Medical Staff

Some donor families feel that they are put under pressure to donate organs by hospital staff, making it very difficult to refuse when the donor is a brain-dead patient. Because the relationship between a doctor and patient (and the patient's family) is a strongly paternalistic one in Japan, the donor family may find it difficult to say no. In such cases, the donor family has no direct motivation for organ donation but feels coerced into it. As a result, they feel mistrust toward not only the medical professionals but also the act of organ donation itself. To make matters worse, they often regret their decision and their grief after the bereavement is deeper and longer.

5. Donor Family's Independent Decision

In one very unusual case, a mother offered to donate her son's organs when she knew that he would die shortly following a serious car accident, even though her son's doctor did not suggest it and she did not know whether her son had an organ donation will or not. When she heard the doctor's explanation of her son's serious situation, she independently and naturally hit upon the idea of organ donation to keep her son's organs alive in recipients' bodies to avoid losing him completely. While we may understand this donor mother's feelings, as a result, she ignored both her husband's and her second son's wishes and broke up the family with disagreements.

THE DECISION-MAKING PROCESS

Many factors also affect the process of deciding to donate a family member's organs. The diversity of donor families gives rise to an equal number of options and dramas.

1. Honoring a Donor's Wish

In one case a donor told his wife that he wanted his organs to be donated and she felt it her duty to bring his wish to fruition. This is an ideal case, in which the organ donation relieved some of the widow's sadness at her husband's death. Nevertheless, the decision might have been affected by the fact that the donor and family member were spouses and thus of an "equal family status": in a parent–child relationship the dynamics can be different, and in fact this donor's mother resisted the idea of organ donation until just before the organs were harvested.

2. One Family Member Leads the Decision

One donor father was influenced by a doctor's suggestion of organ donation because the doctor whispered to him, "There is a way to prolong the death of his daughter" and he seized on the idea as a great one to keep his daughter alive. He decided that he wanted his daughter to live on in others through organ donation rather than allowing her whole body to die and disappear without a trace. He succeeded in persuading the donor's mother; her siblings were too young to make a decision. As a result, this father's opinion became the family opinion through a family meeting and discussion.

3. Family Members Reach a Joint Conclusion

In another instance all family members felt that a donor might have an organ donation will although they did not have any evidence: when watching a TV documentary about organ transplantation with his sister, he had whispered, "If you suffer organ failure, I will donate my organ for you," which both she and other family members heard. The donor's younger sister said, "My big brother is in favor of organ donation for sick people," and all the other family members exchanged their own opinions, with the result that everyone eventually agreed on organ donation.

4. Pressure from Medical Staff

One donor lived with his parents but his father was in the hospital with a serious illness, so the donor's mother had to make the decision to donate on her own without recourse to a family consensus. She felt that the medical staff were over-insistent and forced her to agree to organ donation without allowing her a chance to consider the decision. She felt that the traditional paternalistic attitude of medical doctors toward patients made it difficult for her to say no, but also felt that the doctors cared far more about the recipient than the donor family's grief.

5. Decreasing Donor's Life and Increasing Organ Donation Will

Another donor mother decided on donation by herself without consulting other family members. She could not accept her son's death and was seeking a way to prolong his life: when she knew that he was brain-dead the doctor suggested organ donation and, although initially unsure, the closer his death approached, the stronger her decision to donate became.

ATTITUDES TO ORGAN DONATION

A donation will is one of the most important factors for organ transplantation. It has an impact at every stage, creating awareness before the need arises, informing the decision-making process, and offering assistance and comfort to the donor family after organ donation. Nevertheless, in the urgent situations often encountered in a hospital emergency room, the existence of a donor's will may not be known and the patient's preferences may be unclear. The revised Japanese organ transplantation law of 2010 permits family-presumed consent, allowing the donor family to authorize organ donation in the absence of a donation will. Donor families' narratives again reveal a variety of attitudes to organ donation and subsequent reactions, which give rise to a number of alternative types of decision.

1. Donor's Donation Will

The fundamental principle of organ donation is that of a donor's "gift of life" based on a donation will, but all the organ donation wills mentioned by the interviewees in this research were verbal promises rather than written donor cards. The existence of a donation will makes the difficult situation surrounding the decision to donate much easier for transplant surgeons, recipients, and donor families both before and after surgery: according to my data, donors' donation wills help their families heal after the donor's death. The donation will brings about a physical medical effect for recipients, but also has a psychological influence on the donor family's bereavement, helping the grieving process. According to a specialist funeral director, bereaved families are keen to do anything for the dead family member, so a donor's written donation will is very important and helpful for the bereaved family, whether for or against organ donation.

2. Donor Family's Donation Will

Under the original Japanese organ transplantation law, an individual's organ donation will was a private matter, but the law required both a donor's donation will and the donor family's consent. Difficulties arose, therefore, when the decision to harvest organs had to be made but the donor had not declared that they had a donation will. The revised law permits family-presumed consent, which allows the donor family to make the decision about organ donation: in essence, this creates a joint family donation will rather than an individual donor will, meaning that the human right of self-determination will be overridden in such cases.

3. Individual Family Member's Donation Will

The joint donor family donation will described above reflects the collective opinion of all family members. In the real world, however, it is not always easy to achieve a family consensus, especially in situations involving people without close family members, whose family members may be too young to make a decision, or whose family has a "non-nuclear" structure, including step-parents and children or similar more distant relatives. If a family consists solely of the donor and one other close family member (mother/father, wife/husband, or son/daughter), that individual has a very difficult and weighty responsibility when making the decision about organ donation.

4. Medical Professionals' Donation Will

Fundamentally, medical staff should not lead the decision on organ donation for patients' families to respect patients' autonomy and free will concerning organ donation. Most family members, however, are in a state of distress in the emergency room and the issue of organ donation may not occur to them unless it is brought up by a medical professional unless they themselves have a donor card. Some donor family members are ignorant of—or indifferent to—organ donation and transplantation issues and they need information from staff. Nevertheless, the right of the donor family members to reach their own conclusion must be respected. It is a very sensitive matter, in which the attitude of medical staff must remain entirely professional.

5. A Personal Donation Will

One mother offered to donate her son's organs purely as a means to keep a part of him alive, but with no wish to know about the recipients and their future health or to consider the donation as a "gift of life." One father offered to donate his son's organs because he felt that his son had caused much trouble in his life: the donation was an effort to purify his son and to apologize to the world on his behalf. After the donations, though, this father and mother were both wracked with a sense of guilt and helplessness. He later wanted to know about the recipients' health to check whether they were alive or not, but she refused to be informed of the recipients' condition because if their bodies had rejected the organ or they had passed away it would mean her son's second death.

For a donor family, the existence or lack of a donor's organ donation will is a huge factor affecting their motivation, decision making, and attitude to the donation. In addition, as mentioned above, "family status" is a crucial factor that must be taken into account when considering blood or married relationships in Japan, because recently the way families are constructed has been changing and has diversified. The next section introduces donor families' narratives, paying particular attention to the family status of the donor and donor family member.

DONOR FAMILIES' NARRATIVES

The motives behind a donor family's decision to agree to organ donation are various and complex, and (as seen above) donors' donation wills are a very important factor. The relationships between donors and members of their families are also highly significant: they influence donor families before and after organ donation. In interviews with six donor family members—two fathers, three mothers, and a wife—the differences in narratives of the donor parents and the donor spouse were interesting. While a spouse is connected to the donor by will or love, making their relationship equal, a parent's blood connection to their donor child is a more fundamental and emotional relationship. At times it can be difficult to understand their narratives logically, as they appear to turn metaphors (such as "my child lives in me") into their own reality. In addition, in Japan the family ties between mother and child are generally much stronger than those between father and child.

Against previous expectations, all the donor family members were keen to disclose their motivations for donating organs (I was warned that donor families never talk about their organ donation). Five donor families accepted their doctor's offer of organ donation; another donor mother felt unable to refuse the doctor's request because her son had a brain hemorrhage and was hospitalized: she was afraid—within the context of the strong paternalistic medical world in Japan—that his doctor would become angry and refuse medical care until his death. Three parents and the spouse agreed with existing or assumed donation wills, including a father who, when offered the choice by the doctor, felt that this was an ideal way to allow his daughter to live on as a donated body part. Unusually, one donor mother proposed the donation of her son's organs herself to avoid his "complete" death—so that she felt his organs could live forever with her.

DONOR FATHERS' DECISIONS

The Japanese family system is still rather conservative and family members are not granted the same level of individuality and independence as would be expected in the West. Patriarchy is not as strong in modern Japanese society as in the era before World War II, but its cultural hold still persists, especially in the home. Fathers have high status within the Japanese family, but tend to have minimal involvement in parenting even a sick child in daily life, leaving their children's upbringing to their wives. In addition, Japanese fathers' attitudes are different toward sons and daughters. A son will be brought up with stricter discipline than a daughter, but a father's expectations of pride in a son's future are greater, while he will be mentally prepared to give his daughter away once she grows up.

The Japanese father's traditional role is to work and earn money to support his family members outside the home: the traditional Japanese social system in which "men should be businessman and women should be housewives" is still quite prevalent. Of course the father loves his children, but an attitude of self-restraint is culturally more acceptable than emotional displays. As a result, he may have too little information about his child to make an informed medical decision. Nevertheless, a father is considered a more objective judge of what is best for a child than a mother in Japanese society. He is expected to assume the lead role in the sort of crucial decision-making involved in organ donation, and to take responsibility for the final decision of the family consensus with strength, aplomb, and a lack of emotion, which is an extremely tough challenge to face.

Donor Father Fukuzawa's Decision—Following His Son's Wishes

Donor father Fukuzawa is sixty-two years old, married, high-school educated, and a self-employed businessman. His son died at the age of twenty-three in Sydney, Australia, and the family (including his wife and a younger daughter) decided to donate his kidneys and liver following his brain death in December 1991.

> I knew he had an organ donation will: he was such a guy! What should I say. . . . He would do everything he could for others, even if it meant killing himself. I saw such scenes many times in his life. I really respected my son. But if I said this to my wife and my daughter, I would be putting pressure on them, so I wanted to hear their opinions first. My daughter sparked a discussion about my son's organ donation and she said, "He offered to donate his organs to me if I ever needed one when we were watching a TV program about organ transplantation together at home, so he would want to donate his organs for others." My wife nodded and of course so did I: everyone agreed that organ donation was the right thing to do. We satisfied the will of our son, so he must be happy but . . . after the donation, the media barged into our lives and we became a media circus.

Donor Father Sakamoto's Decision—Missing His Daughter

Donor father Sakamoto is fifty-three years old, married, high-school educated, and a salaried worker. His eldest daughter died at the age of twenty-one and the family (including his wife, eldest son and a second daughter) decided to donate her kidney in September 1997.

> I decided on organ donation because I wanted my daughter to live, even if it was only her organ in someone's body. I didn't want her to die completely . . . she is a missing child: she lives inside a recipient's body. But sometimes, I wonder whether this was my own selfish thought and whether my daughter didn't want to donate her organ. I made her experience pain through the organ harvesting even after she died. I was told, "There is a way to donate organs" by a doctor, so I accepted his offer unquestioningly. Of course, we had a family meeting to make the decision to donate my daughter's organ and my wife agreed with me with no comment. My children (a son and a daughter) who were still students just nodded without saying anything. . . . I want to ask her about the donation and to know her opinion, whether she wanted to donate her organ or not: if not, I want to apologize to her. . . . Was this okay? I need my daughter's forgiveness for donating her organ without her permission! I might have no reply from her but I want to communicate with her. That's my wish.

These two donor fathers' narratives are contrasting: the first is proud of his decision to donate his son's organs but the second has been plagued with guilt at the thought of the judgment he made over his daughter's organ donation. Neither regretted the organ donation at the time, but their motives, the family consensus decision-making processes, and their attitudes were completely different. According to these data, knowing about a child's organ donation can make a donor father proud of the donation; however, a lack of a donation will can lead the donor father to feel serious guilt and self-blame. Surprisingly, twelve years after the initial interview research (in 2002), I had a chance to hear of a transformation in their feelings toward their children's organ donation. Now, the son's donor father feels guilt and regret, along with his wife, whose regret has only grown stronger over the years, while the daughter's donor father now feels satisfaction about the donation as a result of the support of his wife and donor family support groups.

1. Mr. Fukuzawa's motivation was the likelihood of his son's having an organ donation will, while Mr. Sakamoto's was the doctor's suggestion. This phenomenon occurs not only in the father–child relationship but also in the mother–child relationship, but the family patriarchy still present in Japan means that it seems that Japanese fathers feel more guilty than mothers, having had less time to make the decision and therefore feeling less confident in it.

2. The family of Mr. Fukuzawa exchanged their opinions freely and had already talked about the topic of organ transplantation before the accident. It seems this family maintained excellent communication on a daily basis. The family of Mr. Sakamoto appeared to reach consensus but did not openly exchange their opinions, just remaining quiet. One reason is that they had not had a chance to talk about organ transplantation issues until the daughter became a donor candidate; another is that all family members did not live together at that time so they had less chance to communicate regularly.

3. The different attitudes shown are also connected to the different father/son and father/daughter relationships that are reflective of Japanese traditional customs and cultural issues about boys and girls. Mr. Fukuzawa's narrative about his son shows him trying to consider his son as an equal, man to man, while Mr. Sakamoto's about his daughter is more emotional, as an adult to a child. One kidney transplant surgeon said in public, "I would donate all my son's organs if he became brain-dead but I would not donate my daughter's because she is a girl."

DONOR MOTHERS' DECISIONS

While the motives behind mothers' decisions to donate their children's organs are also varied and complex, their reactions tend to be much more emotional and instinctive, often relying on an idea of "maternal sense" rather than rationalism. In Japan, this theory of "maternal sense" still has strong good support, especially from older people and those who live in more rural and isolated areas where traditional beliefs are still very common. A mother's family status in traditional Japanese society tends to be lower than that of the father and does not give her the role of main decision maker. Nevertheless, in modern times this is starting to change—especially in urban areas—as social and family structures are altering in Japan, meaning that the patriarchal system is becoming less prevalent. There are three basic "types" of mothers in Japan: housewife, part-time worker, and career woman, and their roles affect their relationships with their children and husbands.

1. Traditionally, Japanese housewives were expected to stay at home and take care of the children all day. These mothers tend to know their children much better than the fathers, including any specific medical information.
2. Part-time workers stay at home much of the time but also undertake part-time jobs. Their working times may vary but they still usually spend more time at home with their children than their husbands.
3. Recently, Japanese parents' roles have diversified and a new word (*Ikumen*—men who do *ikuji* [childcare]) has been created. Such husbands stay at home and take care of children and do housekeeping while the wife works for a company full time as a career woman. Some career women had jobs before marriage and chose to return to work after they had children. These mothers share the housework, raising and caring for their children with their husbands; as a result they also share information about the children. Some have to work after they have children through other circumstances, such as single, divorced, or widowed mothers. These mothers spend time outside the home from morning to night so they don't spend all day with their children, but they have responsibility for their family and the authority to make family decisions by themselves. They have to make judgments on critical issues like organ donation alone. These mothers essentially take on the status of the father within the family as well as that of the mother.

Whatever a mother's career choices, she is the one who experienced childbirth: as a result, she tends to feel her children's organ donation as a more painful situation than a father. Fathers know and recognize this. One said, "It is a more heartbreaking event for mothers to donate their children's organs than fathers." The relationship between mother and child is much deeper and closer than that between father and child in Japan. The data show that a mother's overall idea of organ donation and her reaction to donating her own children's organs are different. In the former theoretical discussion it is possible to think and behave rationally, but mothers cannot address their own children's organ donation in an objective fashion. They feel and respond emotionally and illogically, because they feel their children's pain vicariously. Mothers' reactions are unique and can be difficult to understand.

Donor Mother Fukuzawa's Decision—Sticking to Her Son's Style

Donor mother Fukuzawa is sixty-one years old, married, high-school educated, and a housewife. Her son died at the age of twenty-three in Sydney, Australia, and the family (including her husband and a younger daughter) decided to donate his kidneys and liver following his brain death in December 1991.

> Death, my own son's death . . . it is so sad . . . there are no words: I can't explain! The only person who could understand would have been through the same experience. Never say to me, "That's sad" or "Poor you" because you never know how sad I am: you won't get it! People say they understand but it is just all words. I was . . . I did the same thing to a friend who lost her child . . . but I wonder whether fathers grieve over the death of sons much more than mothers. My husband was really shocked but we knew about my son's organ donation will so we had no trouble about the organ donation itself. . . . Just sadness . . . more than a sad feeling, I thought I would be broken, that I myself could be destroyed. . . . I flew to Australia and rushed to his hospital and when I saw my son's face, I didn't understand what had happened. It must be a dream: I hoped it was a nightmare. A nurse came to me and gestured: "Cry, cry in my arms." I wouldn't dream of crying in an Australian nurse's arms and she said, "Isn't that sad? I have a son almost the same age, if he becomes brain-dead in a foreign country, I would also be sad and so cry in my arms." I learned that Australian and Japanese mothers are the same. Because of my son's organ donation, I had a chance to share other mothers' feelings even in Australia. Also, when our friends visited and talked about my son's organ donation, they said to us, "That's your son's style," "That's typical of him," or "It's very him, your son!" These phrases make me so happy and heal me best.

Donor Mother Honda's Decision—Ensuring Her Son's Survival

Donor mother Honda is fifty-three years old, divorced, junior-college educated, and an office worker. Her elder son died at the age of twenty

and she decided to donate his kidneys following his death in 1996 without input from her ex-husband or second son.

> When my doctor told me "There is no hope" I asked about organ dona-
> tion because I didn't want to lose everything. I hit upon the idea of
> organ donation and then I informed my doctor; there was no offer from
> the doctor. I just wished to make my son alive in someone else's body
> to avoid his death. Even two kidneys are enough to survive inside
> someone, somewhere. Thanks to organ donation he didn't die, but his
> kidney lives in someone's body, although I had no idea of helping
> someone else with my son's organs at that time. Although he is still
> alive I did not offer the "gift of life" at all: I didn't donate his organs to
> help someone, I just thought of him. After the donation, I had a feeling
> that I hadn't lost everything and that my son survived—he is part of
> me now so we live together. After the donation, he is always inside me,
> so I can always feel him and I'm not lonely anymore. He is a part of my
> body so he is alive with me, that's why he didn't die and we are not a
> bereaved family but a living family. Because I'm always with my son I
> refuse to commemorate the anniversary of his death, but I still celebrate
> his birthday. But if we are called a donor family, and someone was
> saved with my son's organ through the so-called "gift of life," actually
> yes, this was the result, but I had no plan to save someone and was not
> trying to do a good thing. I don't want to hear about other donors . . .
> because I'm afraid to hear about a recipient's death! My ex-husband
> asked the latest status of my son's organs' recipients and we learned
> that one recipient's kidney had failed. If another kidney were to fail in
> the recipient's body, it means that my son had died absolutely. I'm
> scared of that.

Donor Mother Noguchi's Decision—Creating Her Son's "Rebirthable Life"

Donor mother Noguchi is seventy-seven years old, married, educated
in a women's school, and a housewife. Her son died at the age of thirty-
six and with no other family members to consult with she decided to
donate his organs (two kidneys, heart valves, two eyeballs, skin, bones,
and cells) following his heart death from subarachnoid bleeding in No-
vember 1996.

> My son left home as usual and I got a phone call from his office: he had
> had a kind of stroke and I rushed to the emergency room. His doctor
> offered organ donation because my son was still young and fresh and
> his healthy organs could save many recipients. I know that organ dona-
> tions are helpful for critically ill patients but I didn't know my son's
> donation will without his donor card. Also my husband was undergo-
> ing treatment at another hospital and we have only one child so I had
> to make a decision about organ donation alone. I hesitated—I was too
> sad about my son's death to think about organ donation, there was no
> room for me to think about it. However, the doctors and coordinators
> negotiated with me personally and it was an environment where I

could not speak out about my true feelings, so I felt I could not say no. I agreed to organ donation without my son's permission and without talking to my husband, who was resident at another hospital. I was full of sorrow for harvesting my son's organs as his parent without his donation will, when he was given back to me and I looked at his lifeless form! It was an unbearable feeling for a mother to see my son's body with its organs harvested. After the donation there was no news from the recipients who were given my son's organs except one thank you letter. I would really like to know about the recipients—whether they are alive or not. A kidney recipient wrote to me with immense gratitude that she can now live an ordinary life without artificial dialysis. I was so happy that I wrote back to her, but after that I had no contact from her. However, time is the best medicine and time heals everything. And I thought that I could imagine my son's organs living and existing somewhere in this universe. Now, I can wish for the recipients' health and happiness. Organ donation . . . is wonderful for both donors and recipients because both donating and receiving organs is a miracle. It's doubly good . . . it is really a "rebirthable life"! Only lucky people can donate and receive organs.

It is difficult to find common characteristics among these three donor mothers' narratives, as each has such a specific emotional reaction to their son's organ donation. Mrs. Fukuzawa suffered a major trauma with her son's death and her narrative scarcely mentions organ donation: her son's death is by far the biggest issue for her, even now. Mrs. Honda offered her son's organs of her own volition to avoid the feeling that he had died completely, and one of her son's kidneys is still "alive." Mrs. Noguchi was working slowly through the grieving process and found a positive interpretation of organ donation as "rebirthable life" for donors. Again, these mothers' motives, the decision-making processes, and their attitudes were different.

1. Mrs. Fukuzawa's motivation was the likelihood of her son's having an organ donation will, Mrs. Honda's was avoiding her son's "complete" death, and Mrs. Noguchi felt she was pressured into the decision by medical staff. When I interviewed these three very different ladies in 2002, it seemed that the donor mother with the best situation was Mrs. Fukuawa. However, according to my follow-up research, Mrs. Honda and her son's organ recipients have now exchanged friendship, and Mrs. Noguchi has a good relationship with her son's organ recipients through events such as transplant games. Mrs. Fukuzawa, however, still is at home with no chance to communicate with her son's organ recipients and feels very isolated; this indicates that continuous mental healthcare is important for the donor family.

2. All three donor mothers had complicated decision-making processes. All spent more time at home and therefore had more infor-

mation about their children than the donor fathers. Nevertheless, their circumstances and the relationships between them and their children's fathers were key factors. Mrs. Fukuzawa and her husband are a very loving couple and part of a close family, so she could accept her husband's and daughter's opinions easily. In a contrasting situation, Mrs. Honda and her husband were in the process of splitting up (they divorced just after their son's organ donation) and the family was in danger of falling apart, so it was difficult to have a family meeting to gather everyone's opinions. Mrs. Noguchi lived with her son, who was an only child, and her husband was resident in another hospital, making it impossible to have a discussion and reach a family consensus. After their son's brain death just the couple remained of their family.

3. The mother–son relationship is the only one available for consideration in this narrative research, but each family structure was different—the first-born donor son and younger daughter, the elder donor son and younger son, and the only child donor son—so their statuses and roles in their families were also different, affecting their attitudes toward the organ donation. However, the role of mothers and fathers has been changing among young couples in Japan in recent years: this may lead to transformed new relationships between fathers and sons and fathers and daughters. Since World War II, Japan has changed from a traditional country to a more cosmopolitan one in urban areas like Tokyo, but however much medical technology has advanced, old-fashioned traditional Japanese beliefs, cultural customs, values, and concepts of life and death have not changed so quickly within the small country.

DONOR WIFE'S DECISION

A wife's decision to donate her husband's organs provides an interesting comparison with the donor parents' cases to understand how the relationships between blood family and legal family differ or are connected. Her decision-making processes about organ donation were simpler than those of donor parents because husband and wife are connected by marriage—and therefore equal partners—rather than tied by blood in a patriarchal or matriarchal relationship. In fact, in Japan the bonds of marriage are weaker than in the West, because Western marriages are more individual, linking person to person, while Eastern marriages are more collective, linking house to house. Conversely, the parent/child bond seems much stronger in the East, where a child is expected to take over as head of their parents' house and take care of their parents in old age.

The family status of wives in Japan is usually weaker than that of their husbands, but this is not always apparent in organ donation issues. Before World War II, most Japanese wives were housewives who were entirely economically dependent on their husbands. According to tradition in Japan, women should be in the house, raising the children and protecting the household; these values are still prevalent in Japanese society, although in modern times some Japanese wives also have a full-time or part-time job to support the family budget. Nevertheless, most Japanese wives quit work after marriage, feeling forced to choose between a career and marriage. Again, there are three basic "types" of wives in Japan: housewife, part-time worker, and career woman, and again, their role affects their relationships with their husbands.

1. Housewives usually stay at home all day, often because old-fashioned views that this is the appropriate role for a woman are still prevalent among elderly people (including parents-in-law) in the countryside in Japan, and few full-time jobs are still available for women. Most Japanese wives devotedly care for their husbands if they have a serious disease, seeing it as their "mission," and obey their husbands' wills in all matters, including organ donation. However, Japanese society has been changing in recent years, and the Japanese *Ie* [feudalistic family system] has been crumbling, which may lead to greater gender equality in the future, although there appears to be some way to go to achieve this as attitudes are slow to change so thoroughly.

2. Wives who have a part-time job are usually just supplementing their husbands' salaries so they are not independent. Housework is still their main job, so Japanese wives working as part-time employees take care of their sick husbands.

3. Career wives often retain full-time jobs from before their marriages. If their husbands suffer from diseases they have to choose whether to keep up their business and hire a nurse or to quit and take care of their husbands themselves. In the former case they are economically independent of their husbands so they do not need to obey their wishes: they share an equal relationship and can discuss nursing and even organ donation wills when their husbands are ill. But in the latter case they lose not only their careers but also their salaries, making them economically dependent on their husbands. This tends to mean that they show their husbands obedience and give them all decision-making rights. The status of a Japanese wife is strongly connected with economic factors and can be very impermanent.

Because donor wives and their husbands are connected by choice rather than blood ties, it is possible for them to think more rationally about organ donations issues than parents and children. The donor wife stated that losing a child and losing a spouse would be very different (she has a daughter). She mentioned that she was sad about her husband's death but not about the organ donation, especially as her husband had a very clear organ donation will. She saw organ donation as her wifely mission because she could not save her husband from his brain tumor, but she could make his wish come true by donating his organs. She did, however, wonder whether she would donate her own daughter's organs in the same situation. In fact, despite being proud of his decision to donate both before and after the operation, her husband's mother was strongly against her son's organ donation at the moment his organs were harvested: as a mother she resisted emotionally.

Donor Wife Suzuki's Decision—Fulfilling a Wife's Mission

Donor wife Suzuki is forty-three years old, educated in a ballet school in England, and a classical ballet instructor with one daughter. She decided to donate her husband's organs (two kidneys, heart valves, two eyeballs, skin, blood vessels, and trachea) following his death from a brain tumor in December 1998.

> My husband had a donation will and we discussed organ donation daily because he was a brain surgeon and advocated organ donation after brain death. I thought I should support his will, considering both his professional position and his private opinion. Because I couldn't cure his brain tumor, all I could do was make his wish come true as a wife's mission. We had been fighting his brain tumor together and I learned from him how he wanted to live his remaining life and his decision to be an organ donor at the end. I informed his doctor of his donation will when it came to the end of his life and I agreed to the donation in advance in order not to waste his organs and tissues, so his colleagues and I can feel his satisfaction every day! My husband's organ donation went well and helped to steer his colleagues, our family members, and me toward healing our grief at his death. Although my mother-in-law agreed with her son's organ donation decision, she was in a panic and against the procedure at the moment when the surgeon had a chance to harvest the organs. Of course, I was surprised by her emotional reaction but I could imagine her feelings as a mother. If my daughter died and we (my husband and I) agreed with organ donation, maybe I might be upset and scream "No!" irrationally at the moment of organ harvest. For mothers, when it concerns our own children, we lose our ability to think rationally and we can say unreasonable things. This is neither taught nor learnt, but we feel their pain as our own pain.

This donor wife's narrative is completely different from those of the donor parents—it is clearly much less emotionally wrought. While sad from the bottom of heart from her loss, it is a different kind of sadness from that of a mother for her deceased child. She also raises several important points, including the fact that there she feels a great difference between harvesting her spouse's and her daughter's organs. She acknowledges that her husband's organ donation will was a very important element of her decision to donate his organs because she thought that making her late husband's wish come true was a wife's mission. She also recommends discussion of organ donation issues when a couple is in good health, as a precaution. As yet there is no narrative data from a donor husband, but research is continuing.

1. Mrs. Suzuki's motivation was her husband's wish to donate, shown in his donation will and both his professional and private opinions as a brain surgeon and his advocating organ transplantation from brain-dead status. Since she could not cure his brain tumor she decided to try to carry out his wish as a wife's mission. She said, "My husband's death is sad thing but organ donation heals me because it was his wish."

2. To assist the organ donation decision she had her husband's organ donation will. The family consensus was very simple, since the only parties were the donor wife and her very young daughter, but she also asked the donor's mother's opinion, even though they did not live together, and canvassed family opinions from the donor's brothers and sisters and other relatives. Fortunately, all family members respected the donor's organ donation will and the donor wife was relieved that everything went smoothly, as she had heard of other cases where a family member, especially a donor's mother, had decided against organ donation, even when there was a donation will. If she had lived with her mother-in-law the family consensus might have become more difficult because there are often difficulties between wives and their husbands' mothers in Japan.

3. The only spousal narrative so far is from this donor wife, so future research may need to focus on gaining information from a donor husband, because Japanese wives depend on their husbands financially, but Japanese husbands depend on their wives emotionally at home. In addition, this donor couple only had a daughter too young to voice an opinion, but older children's views are also important factors and may affect such decisions. The family statuses of donor wives and husbands and their family members, as well as their varied family structures, may also result in different effects, particularly when the unusual relationship of Japanese mothers- and daughters-in-law is taken into account.

DONATED LIFE

In Japan, the donor family's life is still difficult owing to misunderstandings among the public about organ transplantation; consequently, organ donation is still rare. This means that the number of donor families is lower in Japan than in other countries. Many donor families are isolated from their communities or are criticized by others. Their lives are not proud ones, and they tend to hide the fact that they permitted an organ donation. They also produce their own rational interpretations for the decision. Donor families have faced their family member's death and sought a way to keep a part of the dead family member alive. They have reached the organ donation decision by various routes, often without the donation will of the dead family member. For many, organ donation is a ritual that allows donors to be reborn to their own families through narrative.

Japanese mothers' and fathers' narratives are somewhat distinct, and it is easy to see the difference in the relationship between mother and child and father and child—in other words, between a housewife mother and child and a businessman father and child. When I stayed in the United States, I felt that American mothers spent more time with their husbands than Japanese mothers and less with their children, while American fathers spent more time with their families than Japanese fathers and less with their co-workers.

In the fathers' narratives, a child's sudden death in a car accident is very difficult to accept and they think about many ways to keep their child alive, even just as one kidney. The fathers' stance toward their children is more distanced and their interpretation is more objective. One donor father said, "My daughter lives in someone's body somewhere just like a missing child and I hope that she is fine."

The relationship between Japanese mothers and children can be much closer than in Western countries: Japanese mothers tend to maintain a stronger relationship with their children, even after they have grown up, and sometimes imagine their organ-donating children still inside their own bodies like fetuses. In the mothers' narratives, a child's sudden death is an incredibly difficult event to endure and their shock is beyond imagination. In one example, a donor mother struggled with sadness about her son's death, but she tried to avoid his "complete" death by donating his kidneys to keep him alive inside someone else's body. For her, organ donation was an egoistic choice: she had no plan to save others' lives. At that time she thought she could not have the desire to save or do good things for someone else; she just cared about her son's life and avoiding his death, but her feelings changed gradually to the recognition that her son saved two recipients. She insisted that, as a result, the donation was a "gift of life." Mothers also tend to believe that their child lives on with them and that the mother and child will always be together, one mother even declaring, "My son lives inside me!" Donor families' attitudes to their donations and their lives in terms of the donors are very complex. In some cases, donors can be reborn in donor families' minds as a result of narratives.

According to the data, all donor families feel the same duty toward donors. Parents, in particular, feel they owe a debt to their children, but this brings both positive and negative connotations. When donor families are aware of the donation will of a dead family member they are proud of both this decision and the donor's life in this world. They often also make plans to donate their own organs at the end of their lives to reexperience their family member's donation and to share and feel the pinch of organ harvesting. When the dead family member does not have a donation will, however, donor families feel guilt for allowing the donation and feel they must beg forgiveness. Japanese donor parents who donate their children's organs without a donation will feel especially guilty on behalf of their dead children. As a result, they often also plan to become donors as a way of vicariously experiencing and sharing the painful experience they feel they have inflicted on their children. They think they should volunteer for organ donation to make a sacrifice on behalf of their children who became donors.

REBIRTHABLE LIFE

Narrative data from donor families show that while it is possible to say that the organ recipient's and donor's roles in the transplantation process are different—one giving and one receiving life—both equally continue to live among the concerned parties. Some donor family members are eager to know everything about the recipients, and especially love receiving thank you letters, while some want to know nothing about the recipients, especially since news of a recipient's death would make them feel that the donor had also died. This means that the emerging medical technology of organ transplantation has created not only the new agent of the donor but also a new type of life: "rebirthable life." This is also a new type of agent for concerned parties; it has special power over them.

A donor can be reborn in the donor family's mind through organ donation, but this is an invisible and limitless metaphorical life. The donated organ can live inside the recipient's body as part of their limited biological life, so it will die someday, but the donor's life becomes non-biological and non-existent, created by their family's narrative, so that it can live forever in the donor family's imagination. The donor family accepts that the donor's human life has finished, but the donated organs still have biological life inside the recipients' bodies, so the donor family creates the whole-body image of a new type of family member from the donated organ. The donor can gain an endless life in the donor family's mind and grow stronger through their narratives, day by day.

My tentative conclusion is that "rebirthable life" exists for both organ recipients and donors. This new concept of life is ambiguous, complex, and changeable, even among concerned parties. The recipient's life has changed and his/her organ has been replaced by someone else's, so the recipient's body becomes a hybrid (Lock 2000). In addition, the donor's body is cremated without the donated organ and the donor is legally dead, although his/her donated organ still remains biologically alive. That donated organ can live inside someone else's body until the recipient's death or the donated organ's failure. All donor families are confused by such a life—that is, a mostly dead, partly alive person. But donor families are better able to cope with the loss of a family member with more than just a memory, now that the donated organ is alive inside someone, somewhere. While the concept of "rebirthable life" is a kind of fantasy, donor families depend on the donated organ and evoke the memory of the new whole body of the donor.

Organ transplantation has produced this new concept of "rebirthable life," which exists not only among donor families but is also shared by recipients and transplant surgeons, spreading among concerned parties invisibly but powerfully. New concepts of life, such as "rebirthable life," are necessary to help concerned parties and others to adjust to new medical treatments gradually. Brain and heart death, organ donation, and the existence of endless non-biological "rebirthable life" are new agents produced by this innovative technology.

REFERENCES

Inhorn, M., and Wentzell, E. (2011). "Embodying Emergent Masculinities: Reproductive and Sexual Health Technologies in the Middle East and Mexico." *American Ethnologist* 38(4), 801–815.

Lock, M. (2002). *Twice Dead: Organ Transplants and the Reinvention of Death.* Berkeley: University of California Press.

Yasuoka, M. K. (2004). "Six Patterns of Grieving Processes in Organ-Donating Decision Makers: Narratives from 5 Donor Families." *Challenges for Bioethics from Asia,* Eubios Ethics Institute, New Zealand, 274–281.

———. (2006). "Rebirthable Life: Medical Anthropology Study of the Concept of Life According to Concerned Parties Involved in Brain Death and Organ Transplantation." PhD thesis: Department of History and Anthropology (Medical Anthropology), Graduate School of Letters, Hokkaido University, Sapporo, Japan (unpublished).

FIVE

The Buds of Interrelationships among Concerned Parties

INTRODUCTION

Organ transplantation is one of the triumphs of the emerging medical technologies of the twentieth and twenty-first centuries. It is an innovative medical treatment that has created many new ways to save a patient, including donation, harvesting, replacement, and reception of organs. It has also produced new agents of conventional medicine such as donors, recipients, and donor families. Naturally, it has also generated unexpected problems during its development, and social consensus on organ transplantation has yet to be reached. Of greater concern is the variety of different viewpoints and stances even among concerned parties: their relationships are very sensitive and can give rise to serious emotional tensions. In particular, smoothing the way to mutual understanding in the relationship between recipients and donor families is a very tough process (Fox and Swazey 1992).

Under Japanese organ transplantation law, the recipient and donor family are banned from meeting or contacting each other directly: contact must be made through the Japan Organ Transplant Network (JOTN). If a recipient writes a thank you letter to JOTN, the organization tries to contact the donor family to check whether the members want to accept the letter, which is only sent if the response is affirmative. When donor family members want to find out the status of the recipients of their relative's organs they also have to get in touch with JOTN, which can inform them about the recipients' health condition (including death). Nevertheless, such indirect communication causes stress to both recipients and donor families, creating serious tension between them (Yasuoka 2013).

Initially, transplant surgeons were well aware of the difficulty of recipients and donor families meeting freely. They had even heard of occasions where donor families placed recipients in uncomfortable or even criminal situations with hurtful speech or even by begging for money "in exchange for" the donated organ. Transplant surgeons tried not to come between recipients and donor families but hoped that they would manage to build a relationship of mutual understanding, which might eventually give rise to social consensus about organ transplantation in the country. Recipients, meantime, were afraid that donor families would feel bitterness toward them; they struggled to imagine the feelings aroused toward someone whose survival resulted from a donor's deaths. Donor families also became angry with recipients' attitudes toward the donated organs, not necessarily understanding the magnitude of the changes the surgery had made to their lives, and feeling that their loved ones were not sufficiently acknowledged.

Concerned parties were not satisfied with this situation, and tried to overcome these tensions, coming up with three schemes to resolve the difficulties inherent in the relationship between recipients and donor families.

1. Speak out: surprisingly, recipients and donor families began to speak out independently about their experiences of organ reception and donation at the same time. Recipients and donor families have been trying to listen to each other's words to create a deeper understanding between parties.
2. Thank you letter: this is the only legally permitted way for recipients and donor families to communicate through JOTN. Although some recipients were happy to write thank you letters to donor families, others were hesitant. Conversely, most donor families waited impatiently for a thank you letter but a few refused to receive one.
3. Transplant Games: various organ recipients participate in the national Transplant Games every year and World Transplant Games every other year to build up recipients' physical strength and to increase awareness of transplant medicine in society. These events also invite donor families and transplant surgeons to offer support together (Yasuoka 2006).[1]

DONORS' POWER: CONTROLLING CONCERNED PARTIES

The new treatment of organ transplantation created a new agent in the medical world: the donor. It is difficult for concerned parties to fully comprehend this new agent, since while the donor is usually dead, his or her donated partial organ is still functioning biologically—and thus remains alive—inside the recipient's body. It has become apparent that the power of the donor is extremely strong, far beyond all expectations. This power is invisible but centers on concerned parties, with a web-like hold over transplant surgeons, recipients, and donor families. The reactions to this power vary among the different concerned parties, but many are troubled or unnerved by the feeling that a dead individual has some form of control over them. With recent changes in approaches and attitudes, however, it is possible to trace a change of mood among concerned parties from antagonism to mutual understanding.

In the Japanese traditional medical world, the relationship between doctor and patient still remains strongly paternalistic, but within the new world of organ transplantation a different relationship is emerging. Transplant surgeons have to bow their heads and beg for an organ donation, and their narratives reveal that their positions have moved from dignified authoritarian doctors to mediators between donors and recipients. Organ recipients are just patients who need medical treatment but they have to depend on donations from an organ donor even more than they do on a doctor. Recipient narratives reveal this reliance: "Where there is a donor, there is my life" and "I can't live without a donor!" Donor families explain that they feel they spent their life with the donor so he or she is still alive beside them or even inside them. Many complain that they should be viewed as a donor family and not a bereaved family, because the family member who donated his or her organ is still alive, even though only their organ remains.

Each concerned party is controlled by the donor in various ways and tries to adjust to a new concept of life and death. All feel that their lives are somehow in a different world after organ replacement surgery, organ reception, or organ donation. In particular, the positions of organ recipients and donor families are felt to be completely opposite. Nevertheless, a donor's power over concerned parties works strongly but unpredictably, and not only in negative ways. All concerned parties appreciate donors from their bottom of their hearts. Transplant surgeons feel a mission to harvest organs from donors and place them into recipients' bodies to save their lives, feeling the donor's human love through the donation. Recipients feel a mission to speak out about their organ reception experiences to show the donors' human love for them. Donor families feel a mission to speak out about their family member's organ donation to complete the donor's will.

SPEAKING OUT 1: NARRATIVES OF ORGAN RECEPTION

Under current Japanese transplantation law there is no way for recipients and donor families to communicate directly: recipients even have to send thank you letters to donor families via JOTN. Simultaneously, however, both groups have recently started to speak out about their individual experiences. As a result, donor families have been able to listen to recipients' stories and vice versa.

1. Narrative of a Liver Recipient

Many Japanese liver transplant recipients relied on overseas transplants, receiving organs from brain-dead donors in Australia (most overseas liver transplant recipients went to Australia before 2008, but Australian hospitals are now banned from accepting overseas organ recipient candidates since the Istanbul Declaration). Ai told how she had had huge anxiety and spent many nights alone in Australia waiting for a liver when she was young. She felt that it was import that she, as a recipient herself, should speak out not only for concerned parties but also for those unaffected, in order to try to build social consensus in Japan. She felt a mission to speak out about her own experience as an organ recipient to help ordinary people understand transplantation.

2. Narrative of a Kidney Recipient from a Brain-Dead Donor

Organ donation from brain-dead donors is still rare in Japan, even after the revision of the organ transplantation law. Japanese kidney recipients in particular mostly depend on living donors inside the family circle. Akira, who received an organ from a brain-dead donor in Japan, had tried to hit on a method to show his appreciation to the donor family, but couldn't think of a good way to approach them. He explained that the organ donation had created a new relationship between him and the donor family, even though he did not know who they were, and he also felt a broader connection with other donor families and recipients. He said that he had therefore been working as a volunteer in an association that contributes to promoting organ transplant events. He attended an international Transplant Games event in Spain and brought back some Spanish souvenirs for donor mothers in Japan to inform them about the World Transplant Games and invite them to attend.

3. Narrative of a Kidney Recipient in the United States in 1985

Because of the outcome of the "Wada Case," Japanese organ transplantation was interrupted from 1969 to 1996: kidney recipients relied on living donors and overseas transplants. Hiroshi had no family and no alternative for survival, so he flew to Ohio in the United States in 1985, when cases of overseas transplants were still rare (he was working in the United States at the time). When he left, he asked his doctor what he should do for the donor family to inform them of his happiness and appreciation. He was advised, "Why don't you lead organ transplant activities at home to enlighten Japanese people?" As a result, he began acting as a leader, preparing and promoting events to enable recipients and donor families to speak out about and share their own experiences.

4. Narrative of a Kidney Recipient in the United States in 2008

Japanese organ transplants restarted in 1997, but there are still severe organ shortages. Many recipient candidates still have to rely on overseas transplants, especially aged recipients whose parents and siblings are too old to be donors. Recently, however, thanks to the continuing development of emerging medical technology, even spouses can donate organs rather than donors being restricted to blood relatives. Ken, who had received an organ overseas because of the lack of Japanese donors, started to speak out about the issue to try to increase knowledge among the public. He insisted that organ transplantation is much more wonderful than dialysis, as it means that recipients don't have to depend on overseas transplants because the family circle has now spread to include wider family members.

5. Narrative of a Kidney Retransplant Recipient

Since both dead and living donors can make kidney donations, kidney recipients are sometimes able to undergo retransplantation. Takeshi received his first kidney from his mother (as a living donor) when he was a child and his second from a heart-dead donor after ten years of waiting and undergoing dialysis. He never spoke about his experience after his first transplant, but after his second he began to attend organ donation-related events, seeking a chance to speak out in public about his experience to both donor families and other parties not associated with organ donation. He also drew cartoons and graphic stories to advocate transplantation in the monthly journal of the Japan Transplant Recipients Organization and attended meetings with staff of the journal.

SPEAKING OUT 2: NARRATIVES OF ORGAN DONATION

Donor families have also recently started to speak out about their experiences of organ donation.

1. Narrative of a Son's Organ Donation by the Donor Father

His son had no donor card but had often told Mr. Fukuzawa during his life that he wanted to donate his organs—for example, when he and his younger sister were watching a TV program about organ transplantation, he told his sister tenderly, "I would donate my organ for you if you needed." So when he had a car accident in Australia and became brain-dead, his father and other family members found it easy to decide on organ donation. The whole family flew to the Australian hospital and brought the son's body back to Japan after his death and organ donation. His father became vice president of a donor family club in Japan and often spoke about his experience, saying that he had "no regret about the organ donation" because of his son's donation will, which was his way of helping someone. Although the donor family was overwhelmed with sadness, this was not for the organ donation but because they had lost their loved one.

2. Narrative of a Son's Organ Donation via a Donation Will by the Donor Mother

Mrs. Fukuzawa tried not to speak about her son's organ donation, just about his memory and her deep grief at losing her only son. Nevertheless, she attended a donor family club with her husband to show her support. She stated that she had no regret about the organ donation because of her son's donation will: she had made his wish a reality and was satisfied that she could complete his life the way he chose. When her friends heard about her decision and her son's donation will they said, "Organ donation? That's the sort of generous person your son was: always trying to help others." Their words of admiration were of great comfort to her. With the international organ shortage more donors are needed, but many Japanese people do not want to donate their organs (Yasuoka 2010), which made this donor mother sad and ashamed that more Japanese people do not try to help each other. Her son died in Australia and donated his organs to Australian recipients, but she and her family knew that he wanted to save someone wherever they were in the world. She also claimed, however, that she had thought recently that if she had not known about her son's donation will, she might have been against the donation. Even though her husband and daughter agreed with it, she wondered whether she would have refused, and despite her pride in her son she remained ambivalent about the donation process.

3. Narrative of a Son's Organ Donation via Her Own Decision by the Donor Mother

Mrs. Honda is a very unusual case: she asked for her son's organs to be donated without either his donation will or the agreement of his other family members. She just wanted her son to live, even as two kidneys inside someone else's body. She insisted that her decision was not a "gift of life" and she even refused a certificate of appreciation from the Ministry of Health, Labor, and Welfare. She wanted to speak out about her experience, however, and tried to send notes or articles to newspapers and donor family club journals, but her tone was provocative and she was mostly ignored, although some surgeons were interested in what she had to say. She claimed that her motivation for organ donation was not initially to save the recipients, and stated that all donor families' motivations are different. But she added, "I hope the recipient is in good health now, as my feelings have changed as a result of the 'gift of life!'"

4. Narrative of a Son's Organ Donation through Medical Staff Recommendation by the Donor Mother

Mrs. Noguchi's son did not have a donor card and she was so upset by his sudden brain death that she could not decide easily on organ donation by herself. She felt that her son's doctor forced her to agree to the donation and that a coordinator who later joined the medical staff also gave her no opportunity to say no. Eventually she accepted the donation, but she regretted the decision when her son's body was returned to her with its changed appearance and she felt she needed to apologize to him. Afterwards, however, she had a chance to meet some recipients and the new idea that her son's organs and tissue were alive somewhere in the universe hit her. She came to feel that the fact that his organs saved someone somewhere was indeed a wonderful thing. Although she was not keen to talk in public she joined a donor family club and wrote articles and notes. She also gave talks and wrote poems about her donor son for her haiku club, as well as attending the Transplant Games and presenting medals to recipients.

5. Narrative of a Daughter's Organ Donation by the Donor Father

Mr. Sakamoto's daughter had a car accident and became brain-dead; she was rushed to the hospital. Her doctor told him that there was a way to avoid his daughter's death with organ donation. All his family members agreed with the organ donation decision but he was later asked how much money he received from it, which gave him a great shock. He felt the need to apologize to his daughter and he suspected that she might hold a grudge against him because of his action. He was looking forward to meeting some organ recipients and seeing them in health, but he also felt anger and sadness, giving way to tears and saying, "I am happy to see recipients in good health but I can't help feeling jealous. . . . Why isn't my daughter here?" He learned that his reactions to recipients contained both rational and irrational emotions, appreciating their health through science but feeling the loss of his daughter even more strongly. He joined a donor family club and began to speak out about his experience, first just within the club but gradually also on the radio and TV.

6. *Narrative of a Husband's Organ Donation by the Donor Wife*

Mrs. Suzuki learned of her husband's donation will while they were battling his illness from a tumor together and she agreed with his thinking and respected his donation will. She became vice president of a donor family club and was invited to give lectures at meetings and educate other people, as well as publishing a book about the donor family. She said that organ donation healed her sadness because it was her husband's decision. This narrative stimulated other donor families; some resented her speaking out as they felt she portrayed only the positive and none of the negative implications of organ donation, but she was aware that there is a great difference between organ donation with a donation will and without, and that her situation was different from some others.

FEELING THE DONOR'S POWER FROM DIFFERENT PERSPECTIVES

All concerned parties reveal that they feel the donor's presence as an invisible force, powerful enough to have some control over them, although the various categories of concerned parties have different perspectives on this power. It is thus difficult for recipients, donor families, and transplant surgeons to understand each other's positions and their own rationally, and to share with each other what the donors' power means to them. In addition, the power of the donor has been getting stronger among some donor families and recipients and weaker among others. The next section attempts to introduce some of these perspectives.

1. *Feeling the Donor's Power by a Heart Transplant Surgeon*

The heart transplant surgeon has one of the strongest roles concerning the donor, donor family, and recipient's life directly by harvesting the donor's beating heart. Brain death is legally categorized as human death in Japan so a Japanese heart transplant surgeon doesn't have to worry about the legalities of the brain-dead donor's life and death, but is nevertheless aware that the donor's heart is still beating, which is a sign of life. Dr. Tanaka reported, "Brain death is human death and I can save a recipient so I have to do it . . . but I can't help having bitter feelings." A heart surgeon must be calm and collected in the operating theatre but organ harvesting still provokes an emotional response.

2. *Feeling the Donor's Power by a Kidney Transplant Surgeon*

Kidney transplant surgeons often say that kidney transplants are different from other transplant operations, such as heart and liver, which have a higher risk of fatality. They insist that kidney transplants offer improvement to a patient's quality of life but do not in fact save lives.

Nevertheless, all surgery carries some risk and even kidney transplants put both a living donor's and a recipient's life in danger to a greater or lesser extent. The kidney transplant surgeon also has to meet a living donor and recipient within the same family circle, adding another kind of pressure to the role. Recently, thanks to the development of emerging medical technology, organ retransplantation has become possible, increasing the number of possible donors per recipient, and thereby increasing the guilt a kidney transplant surgeon may feel when harvesting an organ from a living person who would not otherwise need surgery, thereby placing the donor's life and health in some danger. Surgeons conduct regular study meetings with recipients and pharmaceutical companies to inform and educate them about organ transplantation and try to build understanding about the process.

3. Feeling the Donor's Power by an Overseas Kidney Recipient

When he received a kidney in the United States in 1985, before the organ transplantation law was established in Japan, Hiroshi said that he didn't know anything about the donor: it was probably an American donor, but he had no information about the gender, race, age, and so on. All he could do was pray for a donor when he went to bed every night in Japan (he passed away a few years ago but he kept praying for his American donor every night from 1985 to his death). Afterwards, he said, "I can only feel my donor in the moment, when I am praying for his peaceful sleep in heaven: I appreciate my donor every night and I work as hard as possible to advocate activities in the daytime. I wonder whether someday my donor will forgive my selfishness, because when I was waiting for an organ in the United States, it means that I was waiting for someone's death in order to survive."

4. Feeling the Donor's Power by a Kidney Retransplant Recipient

Takeshi received a kidney from his mother when he was a child, but did not appreciate the donation or take care of himself, so the organ failed within a year. He went back on dialysis again and waited for his second donated organ for ten years, when he was very lucky to receive another kidney from a heart-dead donor. He said that when he received this retransplantation he felt appreciation for it after waiting for ten years. This appreciation stimulated his thoughts for his first donor—his mother—and he felt guilty about his first donation and lack of appreciation at that time, creating very complex feelings toward his first donor. His retransplantation evoked his first transplantation and he felt both donors and their love.

5. *Feeling the Donor's Power by Donor Fathers*

Japanese men culturally and traditionally tend to control their expressions of emotion in public. Japanese fathers naturally feel strongly about their sons or daughters, but they don't talk about their organ donor children as easily as Japanese mothers do. They also tend to feel more emotional toward their daughters than their sons (to whom they have a much cooler attitude). Organ donation by their children is a new experience for most and they tend to speak about it in some puzzlement. Mr. Fukuzawa said that he felt his son pushing him back and saying, "Dad, I helped a recipient, so you should do something for people too." As a result he joined and worked at the donor family club and felt proud of his son. Mr. Sakamoto explained that he feels that his daughter is living somewhere inside the recipient's body, just as if she were married to someone and living away from home. He still wonders whether it was all for the best or not the right result for her.

6. *Feeling the Donor's Power by a Donor Mother*

Japanese donor mothers are much more emotional than donor fathers concerning their organ donor children, but their narratives about their donor sons and daughters reveal opposing reactions and feelings: they demonstrate much more variety than those of donor fathers. Donor mothers also feel confident that they know more about their children than the fathers as childcare "experts." Although Japan is a modern country in many ways, Japanese society is still firmly based on traditional customs and values and the social system has a long way to go to catch up with notion of women's equality. In the last generation, women had to marry after they turned twenty-five years old and were expected to stay at home to do housework for their husband and children. In modern times, women have attained education and jobs but are still expected to take the burden of looking after the household and taking care of children, just as in previous generations.

1. Mrs. Suzuki spoke extensively about the son she had lost, but did not describe him as a donor. For her, it was the son's death and not his organ donation that was the biggest issue in her life. She insisted that if she had not known about his donation will she would have disagreed violently with the donation, no matter what her husband and daughter might have said.

2. Mrs. Noguchi felt her donor son with her every day but her feelings about his donation changed when she met and talked to recipients directly. She came to feel strongly that her son saved many people as a donor and this gave her great pride in his action and helped her to accept his death. She felt that the donor is present inside the recipients, communicating equally with the donor fami-

ly and recipient, so she tried to make contact with recipients at public events. She commented that both donors and recipients are lucky because not all dead people can donate and not all recipient candidates receive organs.

3. Mrs. Honda unusually offered her son's organs for donation by herself to avoid his "complete" death. She wanted to feel that her son was inside the recipients' bodies every moment somewhere; she therefore refused to receive updates on the recipients' conditions because if they passed away, it would mean her son's death.

7. Feeling the Donor's Power by a Donor Wife

Mrs. Suzuki's feelings toward her husband were more rational than those of parents, and she knew him well. She explained that her case was unusual, since fortunately his other family members agreed with her decision to donate and everything went well. She felt the donor's presence strongly when she met recipients in good health, and was glad that her husband had helped them. This was a great comfort to her and she felt happy about the donation—that his donation will saved someone and that she could complete her wifely mission through it. She considered her husband's death and his organ donation absolutely separate: she was devastated by his death but his organ donation helped to heal her because she satisfied her husband's desire to donate. Nevertheless, she commented that, "I love my husband and I am sadder than I can describe but organ donation was his wish so I did it as a wife's mission. But I wonder whether I would be able to donate my own organs or those of my daughter." She continued: "A married couple is tied together by reason but a parent and child, especially a mother and child, are tied together by stronger and less rational feelings."

The next section introduces another promotion of communication between the recipient and donor family, paying attention to the specific concerned parties' dilemma.

DONORS' PRESENCE: PROMOTING COMMUNICATION

Under Japanese organ transplantation law, contact between recipients and donor families is prohibited, with the exception of a thank you letter, which recipients are encouraged to write to donor families through JOTN rather than directly. It is assumed as a matter of course that recipients should write a thank you letter to the donor family: they were given organs by the decision of both the donor and the donor family to donate, and in general, a donor family is happy to receive the letter. Nevertheless, things are rarely so simple, and there are various issues between recipients and donor families that cause concerned parties to struggle with the thank you letter.

It is usually recognized that a recipient should naturally write to thank the donor and donor family and show appreciation for the donated organ, but most recipients do not do so. Recipients' narratives reveal that, even though they received the "gift of life" of organ donation, a wide barrier exists between a recipient and a donor or donor family to say thank you so frankly and cheerfully. The structure of these barriers varies, as every recipient has a different reason for hesitating to write, including both external and internal factors such as language barriers for overseas organ transplant recipients and *Ie* [the feudalistic family system in Japan] for recipients from Japanese donors.

People (especially organ recipients) also assume that all donor families will be happy to receive a thank you letter from a recipient; again, this is not always the case. Their reasons are also complex and involve a variety of external and internal factors. Some donor families hope for a thank you letter to inform them whether their family member's organ saved someone but some have complex feelings about receiving one from a recipient who was given their dead family member's organ. Some refuse to accept the letter to avoid finding out possible bad news about the recipient, such as if they have suffered organ rejection or even death. The motivation behind the decision to donate their loved one's organs is a very important component of the donor family's acceptance of the donor's death and their assessment of the organ donation is strongly connected to this. Their grieving processes are also linked to their daily lives, whether living openly as a donor family or pretending in public that they have had no involvement with organ donation.

THANK YOU LETTER 1: WRITING A THANK YOU LETTER

The thank you letter via JOTN is the only legally permitted communication between recipients and donor families. JOTN's ideal scenario is that a recipient writes a thank you letter to a donor family, which is happy to receive it as an acknowledgement of the precious "gift of life." The real situation, however, is more unpredictable.

1. "I Won't Write because of the Shame of Being a Recipient"

Satoshi hid all his personal information to keep his organ reception from a brain-dead donor secret. He was a very well-mannered individual and appreciated his donor but he had no will to write a thank you letter. He was an only son, living with his parents, so in total three people knew about his organ reception. He insisted, "I am a nuisance to our family. I'm the family's shame: organ reception from a brain-dead person is taboo so it must be kept secret forever and I will carry the tale to the grave. That's why I won't write a thank you letter."

2. "I Won't Write because I Would Not Want to Receive a Letter"

Hana explained that she did not write a thank you letter because she felt that if she were part of a donor family she would not want to receive one. "Before organ reception I thought that recipients should write a thank you letter to the donor family as simple good manners, but when I received my organ I hesitated. When I imagine my donor family's feelings, of course they can't forget their family member's donation, but people's grief can gradually fade over time. If I wrote to them there is a risk that it would re-open old wounds about the donor's death and the painful issues surrounding organ donation. . . . I suspect that it is kinder for my donor family to give them some space, since I don't know their true thoughts about the donation."

3. "I Won't Write: What Should I Write?"

Akira did not write a thank you letter to his donor family at all, even though he had many chances to meet other donor families. He was extremely active as a leader of an association for organ recipients for a long time, trying to create opportunities for recipients to mingle with donor families with his recipient fellows. In an ironic twist, the more he met donor families, the more he knew the depth of their grief and the various difficulties they faced and he felt less able to write. This made him more confused than ever about what he should write in a thank you letter and whether he should write to the donor family or not, because he understood the possibility that the donor family might not want to hear from him at all.

4. "I Won't Write because I Have Two Donors"

Takeshi recipient had two donors—his mother and a cadaveric donor—but did not write a thank you letter to either of them. He said, "I have no idea. . . . I can't imagine how and what the donor family is thinking about me at all. My first donor was my mother, so of course I really appreciate her and her sacrificing love, but we live together, so writing a thank you letter to her it is not appropriate! I try to show my appreciation with a present or something on her birthday instead. But the second donor family . . . what should I write to them? I can't imagine that they are really expecting me to." He told his tale sadly.

5. *"I Want to Write to Communicate with My Donor"*

Ai taught herself English in order to write a thank you letter to her Australian donor family. She was thrilled with her achievement, and the donor's family was happy to receive her letter. After receiving a liver from a male brain-dead donor, she felt she was sharing her life with him. In fact, only a partial section of his liver was present in her body, but she felt she owed her survival entirely to the support of his organ and his loving donation will. "I speak to him all the time from morning to night. Whenever I make a decision I ask and obey his opinion. Someday I want to be a donor when I complete my life, just like my donor."

6. *"I Had to Write Anonymously"*

Hiroshi received a kidney in the United States before overseas transplant became popular in Japan, at a time when he was working in both the United States and Japan. Since his English was good he wanted to write a thank you letter to offer his appreciation. He was cautioned by medical staff, however, and was given no further information about his donor, such as gender or race, other than that it was an American. In addition, he was prohibited from using his own name in the letter so that he would not be recognized as Japanese. He was forced to hide his name and nationality in his letter, even in 1985 in the United States, a less traditional country than Japan, and was unable to write what he had planned. His experience shows the sensitivity and tact required for donor families globally.

7. *"I Couldn't Write until after a Marathon"*

Ken did not write a thank you letter initially, although he had planned one. His letter would be in English, which meant that he needed a translator. He had tried to write as soon as possible while he was waiting in hospital for the organ but once he became a recipient he changed his mind: he started to worry about the donor family's feelings and couldn't write at all. He wondered whether his donor family thought their recipient was also American, and whether they would be disappointed if they found out that they had saved someone Japanese. Eventually, he decided to complete the Tokyo marathon; this gave him a great reason to write, even as a foreigner, since he was now well enough after his transplant to run a marathon.

THANK YOU LETTER 2: RECEIVING THE THANK YOU LETTER

Just as some organ recipients were hesitant to write and show their appreciation, donor families also described their complex feelings toward a thank you letter.

1. *"I Had Nothing from the Recipients but Don't Really Need It"*

Mrs. Fukuzawa, whose son donated organs in Australia, said that she received no thank you letters from the recipients or their families. "The International Committee for the Red Cross or something sent us a small note, that's all. My son had an accident and became brain-dead in Australia and donated to plural recipients, but we heard nothing from any of the recipients. Maybe [Australian government authorities] think that a small note is good enough for the Japanese. We don't need anything else though, as long as my son's precious donation will was completed! I have no room to care about the recipients; since my son saved some Australians, he must be happy enough."

2. *"The Letter Is My Family Treasure"*

Mr. Sakamoto showed me a *Tokomoma* [an alcove in a traditional Japanese room where art or flowers are displayed] and pulled out a box containing valuables. At the top of the box was a letter. He said, "Please read it for my daughter [the donor]." It was a thank you letter from a kidney recipient and her updated information, handwritten rather than typed, which is seen as more precious in Japan. He explained, "Whenever I read this letter, we can feel my daughter is really helping someone and living inside someone's body, even just as one organ, somewhere in Japan. My daughter was born and existed in this world and died but her one kidney is alive and is supporting this letter writer's life. This is our family treasure." He continued: "All our family members have different feelings . . . so we have never talked about the letter in detail, but we are all happy to receive this handwritten letter and keep it in this treasure box. This letter is a part of my daughter, and proof of her life. I am still so sad about my daughter's death, and may be forever, but this letter is a joy of her left for us. Even just one letter can exchange various feelings as a sacred tool of commutation."

3. *"I Don't Need a Letter"*

Mr. Fukuzawa, whose son donated his organs in Australia, insisted that organ donation is a natural thing as a human being when I interviewed him in 2002. He did not receive a thank you letter, but said, "Who can write a thank you letter in Japanese from Australia? Organ donation is very humane behavior and my son had a donation will for people who are struggling with disease. The sad thing for me is that there are many Japanese people waiting for a donor in Australia, a foreign country. But many Japanese people don't want to donate their own organs—they want to be given organs but not to donate: it's shameful!" Twelve years later, I heard from one of his friends that he regretted his son's organ donation and had quit the donor family club in 2014. This shows how much donor families' feelings are changeable and may fluctuate unpredictably.

4. "I Refused to Receive a Thank You Letter"

Mrs. Honda made her own decision to donate her son's organs: because she strongly did not want to lose her son, she tried to think about how to avoid his death and came up with the idea of organ donation to keep his biological activity alive inside a recipient's body. She recognized that this would avoid her son's "complete" death for her, but she did not see it as a "gift of life" and refused to accept any thank you letters. She was also afraid that if the letter included updates on the recipients' health conditions, such as the donor's organ failure, it could mean that her son's organ had died, and thus he would have died "completely."

5. "I Wrote Straight Back to the Recipient"

Mrs. Noguchi, whose son donated multiple organs and tissue, felt that she was forced to agree to the donation by medical staff. Afterwards, she blamed herself and felt she needed to apologize to her son every day. One day, she received a thank you letter from a kidney recipient, thanking her for the organ donation and informing her of the recipient's current good health without dialysis. The donor mother was so happy that she wrote back through JOTN. Unfortunately, she could not continue to communicate by letter, but the first letter made her stop blaming herself and helped her to feel that her decision to donate her son's organs was not wrong. Although he was dead he had saved the recipient, and this fact comforted her. She told her son "You did a good thing for other people." The thank you letter was the best medicine for her.

6. "It Wouldn't Make Any Difference to Me"

Mrs. Suzuki and her late husband, who had a donation will, had had a lot of time to discuss organ transplant issues during his illness (actually, her husband was a brain surgeon and he did determine brain death by himself). She received a thank you letter after donating her husband's organs, and was pleased to hear about the recipient's good health, but said that receiving the thank you letter did not matter to her: "If recipients want to write, I'm happy to receive it, that's all." Her philosophy was that organ donation should happen automatically and not be of such special status that a letter is necessary.

THANK YOU LETTERS SPANNING GRATITUDE AND GRIEF

As shown in the narratives above, it should not be assumed that recipients should find it easy to write to donor families or that the families will be happy to receive a thank you letter. Concerned parties tend to speak more about negative attitudes to writing and receiving thank you letters than positive ones, and the feelings aroused by the letters are much more complex and varied, with deep emotional implications, than might have been thought. It seems, however, that the easier it is to exchange thank you letters, the greater the hope of concerned parties grasping the buds of mutual understanding.

1. Sharing Joy at the Recipient's Life

The most valuable topic recipients aim to describe in a thank you letter is the joy that they have survived thanks to the donation and recipients strongly feel that they want to tell to donor family how happy they are. This honest emotion may logically make the donor family happy on the recipient's behalf, but may also stimulate difficult and complex feelings toward the donor. Especially at the early stages of organ donation, donor families feel their own grief above the recipients' joy of survival.

2. Appreciating the Donor's Life and Death

A recipient's biggest motivation for writing a thank you letter is the urge to voice his or her appreciation for the donor directly. The donor's organ has led to the recipient's survival and better health, but there is no way to communicate with the dead person: the recipient can only write to the donor family. This gives rise to complex feelings because the recipient's life results from the donor's death and the donor family is now bereaved. Therefore, recipients often hesitate to show their appreciation—not because they lack gratitude for the joy of being alive with the donor's organ, but because the donor family is grieving for a family member's death. It is an ironic but unavoidable fact that while the donation of an organ represents humanity and love between the donor and recipient, the donor's death simultaneously puts a barrier of grief between the recipient and donor family.

3. Feeling Indebted to the Donor Family

Recipients feel appreciation toward donors but also feel indebted to donor families because they made the decision to donate their family member's organ. Because organ transplant treatment depends on organ donation, the concerned parties cannot avoid the donor's death, and recipients can find themselves feeling guilty that in some sense they were hoping for the death of someone's loved one in order that they might live. The serious tension between recipients and donor families initially made it difficult for them to reach any mutual understanding, but both parties have been trying to get to know each other and understand each other's different perspectives. A thank you letter may include both joy at life with the donor's organ and the recipient's indebted feelings to the donor family.

4. Valuing the Donor's Life and Donor Family's Decision

Remarkable changes take place in an organ recipient, both physically and mentally, between being a candidate for an organ and a recipient (although the degree of change varies depending on whether the donor is dead or living). Candidates think about a donor's organ or a donor but not about the donor's family members. After the donation, however, they have to establish a human relationship with the donor family: there is no way to show their appreciation to the donor directly but only to the donor family via a thank you letter. For a recipient, the donor's life is extremely precious and has a value too high to describe, especially to the family that has lost such a precious member.

5. Treasuring the Donor's Life

As recipients undergo the change from candidate to recipient, they learn to treasure not only the donor's organ but also the donor's life, far more than had been understood. Donor families also find that the organ donation process evokes strange and changing feelings toward the donor. In addition, transplant surgeons have come to change their own attitudes as medical doctors and recognize themselves as mediators between donors and recipients. Organ donation, harvesting, and replacement are unique matters for each concerned party and reveal the existence of the donor's life in new ways. Concerned parties' narratives show the power of the donor's life over them, despite its apparent end. This awe-inspiring and wonderful phenomenon shows that human life is perceived as incredibly precious and irreplaceable from all the parties' perspectives.

6. Feeling Ambivalent Emotions

Various emotional dilemmas can be aroused by a single thank you letter and there are as many different ambivalent feelings as there are thank you letter writers. Initial research showed hopeless tensions between recipients and donor families, as they found themselves bound up in negative emotions toward each other rather than considering themselves purely the sender and receiver of an organ. As both sides have begun to recognize each other's strength of feeling and to notice the immense value placed on the donor by recipients and donor families, however, the situation is slowly starting to improve, as all parties begin to build mutual understanding.

1. Surprisingly, most recipients did not write thank you letters to the donor family, despite their gratitude for the organ, often because of the difficult situation of having received an organ from the donor but needing to write to a grieving donor family.
2. Unexpectedly, some donor families did not care about receiving a thank you letter at all; others viewed the letters either positively or negatively, eagerly awaiting or refusing to accept them. Such ambivalent assessments and feelings revealed by their narratives show that donor families' reactions cannot be assumed and should be taken into consideration. It should also be borne in mind that even within one family the members may hold various opinions.

7. Receiving Confirmation of an Organ's Survival

Mrs. Honda explained why she adamantly refused to accept a thank you letter from her son's organ recipients. She donated both her son's kidneys after his death in a car accident and her husband asked JOTN about the results. They were told that one recipient had died already, but the other was fine. This meant that one of her son's kidneys had also died and that only one was still alive, so the donor mother became very worried about the remaining organ, which she felt represented her son's remaining life. She and her husband divorced and she moved to the town where she had lived with her son when he was at school, moving away from her relatives. She explained that if she received more letters from JOTN and they told her of the death of another recipient, all her son's life would also have gone from her. The functions of a thank you letter can thus be seen to be incredibly complicated, showing the numerous issues surrounding organ replacement.

The next section describes newly created events designed to nurture mutual understanding between recipients and donor families as well as transplant surgeons, tracing the unique processes with which they struggle as a result of organ transplantation.

DONORS' EXISTENCE: CONSTRUCTING
INTERDEPENDENT RELATIONSHIPS

The Japanese organ transplantation law prohibits private meetings between recipients and donor families, but transplant surgeons and the
Japan Transplant Recipients Organization have set up a new event: the
Transplant Games. These take place annually in Japan; the World Transplant Games take place every other year. The event's primary aim is to
improve the health of organ recipients through sport, but it is also a
precious annual occasion at which concerned parties can get together and
share their feelings toward donors. Transplant surgeons join the games
and encourage recipients to attend; they also invite donor families. It is
thus a unique opportunity for all concerned parties to meet and communicate directly in public. This has created a movement from isolation to
inclusion and opened an avenue of dialogue.

While all recipients feel strong appreciation toward both donors and
donor families, they do not know what the donor families may think
about them: they may be deeply tempted to know but they cannot. In
addition, many recipients have no idea how they should address donor
families: should they start with hello or thank you? They may feel a
mixture of fear, guilt, and reticence, and the event can provide a stressful
challenge. These anxieties can make recipients avoid meeting donor families directly at the Transplant Games. Such complex feelings and emotional obstacles have led to a prevention of mutual understanding for a
long time, but recipients need to gain the opportunity for human contact
with donor families and the Transplant Games are a great opportunity to
develop this naturally through sport.

Most donor families are sincerely interested in recipients but do not
know how to get into touch with them. Some take care not to give the
impression of patronizing recipients, while others wait for recipients to
say something to them and are hesitant about approaching them. Some
donor families attend the Transplant Games as spectators and some as
players of sports. By watching and playing sports with recipients they
can learn about each other, noticing similarities and understanding their
links through their donors' existence: when meeting recipients, donor
families can share their feelings about donors. At the same time, both
sides can begin to understand that while recipients need donors to save
their lives, donor families need recipients' bodies to preserve the donors'
living organs.

TRANSPLANT GAMES 1: A MEETING PLACE FOR PRECIOUS LIVES

All concerned parties—transplant surgeons, recipients, and donor families—can get together during the Transplant Games. They feel the do-

nors' existence together simultaneously as medical contributors, partial organ carriers, and life-savers.

1. Donor and Organ Mediator

Transplants surgeons describe themselves as matchmakers between recipients and donors, giving donors' organs to recipients with medical technology and thus giving a donor's love to save someone's life. The existence of donors succeeded in breaking down the traditional Japanese paternalistic relationship between doctors and patients and set transplant surgeons in a new position of mediator between donors and recipients. Dr. Sasaki described how moving he found it at the Transplant Games, seeing the standing ovation given to donor families by recipients and feeling pride in his part in the transplantation process that enabled him to be present at such an emotional sight. At the same time, surgeons can check their recipient patients' medical progress. One noted that his patient "attended last year in a wheelchair; surprisingly, he was running this year. Even though he came in last, that is the sign of a great recovery!"

2. Donor and Organ Recipient

Thanks to donated organs, recipients can survive with transplanted organs within their bodies. They naturally feel deep appreciation for both the donor of the organ and the donor family that decided to donate, but their life-changing experience also leads to unpredictable thoughts and emotions too. They may feel such strong appreciation of their donors that they believe they must obey the donors' wishes in order to avoid their bodies rejecting the organs. Although the donors died, the transplanted organs are still alive in the recipients' bodies and the recipients depend on the organs' vitality, thereby creating a subservient relationship to the donors' organs, and indeed the donors. One recipient described how she could not stop her tears of appreciation not only for her donor but for all donor families during the Transplant Games opening ceremony, and felt the strength of the donor's organ within her, giving her life.

3. Donor and Donation Decision Maker

For donor families, the decision to donate a loved one's organs is one of the biggest and most difficult they will ever make, especially if there is no donation will. With a clear donation will, the decision is somewhat easier and they can slightly separate the donor's death and organ donation; it also helps them feel that they are making the deceased donor's wish a reality. Without a donation will, however, donor families have to be the sole decision makers and this experience can make their grieving processes longer and harder. One donor mother described her feelings on entering the Transplant Games to a standing ovation for donor families. She saw one recipient crying and said to her, "Thank you! Please take care of my son's organ." At that moment she felt emotionally connected to all recipients and concerned parties to organ transplantation.

TRANSPLANT GAMES 2: A SPACE TO FEEL DONORS' LIVES

All three categories of concerned parties to organ transplantation feel the donors' existence and emotional accessibility among them during the Transplant Games.

1. Constructing a Sense of Togetherness

Transplant surgeons and their organ recipient patients still maintain a traditional paternalistic relationship after organ transplantation, but recipients also become obedient to their donors, doubling their subservient relationships. The actual relationship between recipient and donor is not fully understood, but it appears that the donor's control and recipient's subservience are tied not only to medical issues but also to their psychology, as recipients feel that they share their lives with donors. Dr. Tanaka said: "I always attend the Transplant Games, playing sport not only with my patients but also with unknown recipients from further afield. . . . Donor families also join our games as players and watchers: who could have imagined donor families, recipients and transplant surgeons all participating in sports together? It truly warms my heart to see it."

2. Sharing Gratitude among Organ Mediators and Receivers

The relationship between doctor and patient is still strongly paternalistic in Japan, but organ transplant treatment has worked to break this traditional relationship: doctors beg patients for organ donations and transplant surgeons and recipients wait together, longing for organs from donors to complete the surgery, which they also go through together. Transplant surgeons' and recipients' appreciation for donors is thus very strong and they share an equal relationship of gratitude as their roles transform from doctor and patient to organ mediator and recipient. Transplant surgeons and recipients join together to welcome donor families to the Transplant Games to show their appreciation to donors. One recipient said, "Some recipients come to the Transplant Games to say thank you to donors together with others . . . we recipients, donor families, and transplant surgeons have shared a unique experience and we can feel the donors together here at the Transplant Games."

3. Donation Decision Makers and Recipients Feeling a Donor's Life

Organ donation creates brand new points of contact between donor families and recipients. At first they seem to be on opposite sides and may feel that serious issues lie between them, but at the Transplant Games they have an opportunity to meet each other and think together about donors and donors' lives. As a result, they may come to realize that both donor families and recipients care deeply about donors. One donor mother said, "I feel that all recipients hold my son's organs: it's not an issue of one person to another. Organ transplantation binds all donor family members' donated organs to all recipients, all donors, and all transplant surgeons as the concerned parties. We are all proud of the donors, care about recipients' health and hope for medical developments for transplant surgeons. We are pioneers and miracle-makers in this world with the donors' precious human love."

TRANSPLANT GAMES 3: A FORUM TO RECOGNIZE INTERDEPENDENT RELATIONSHIPS

Despite the legal prohibition on private meetings between recipients and donor families in case trouble arises, all recipients are interested in their own donors and many want to meet donor families. All donor families also care about recipients and many want to meet them; most donor families feel that their family member's organ is still alive in a recipient's body so they want to meet "recipients" as a group, although not necessarily the particular individual recipient of their loved one's organ. Transplant medical staff also try to be present at the Transplant Games in order to bring these parties together in non-threatening surroundings.

1. Receiving "Biological Life" from the Donor's Organ

Recipients who receive transplanted living organs from brain-dead donors may feel guilt that they were waiting or even hoping for the donors' death. Receiving "biological life" is not as simple as it might seem and recipients may feel that they receive not only the organs but also the donor family's expectations. For some, organ donation is not only the "gift of life"—it may bring other responsibilities, which some recipients can accept as their mission but others cannot. Ai stated, "We donor family and recipients share the donor's life: recipients can't live without the donors' organs but the donors' organs also can't live without recipients' bodies. This made me realize that we can share . . . a feeling of connected fellowship with no barriers of language, race, religion, or borders. We are recipients now but someday I want to be a donor when I complete my life."

2. Showing Appreciation for the Donor Family

The Transplant Games are not just a sporting event; they have various meanings for all concerned parties. The current Japanese organ transplantation law offers no opportunity for recipients to say thank you directly to donor families. Some recipients lack public speaking skills or struggle to write thank you letters, but the Transplant Games provide precious opportunities for concerned parties to communicate through playing sport together in the daytime or eating and drinking together at night. The period of the Transplant Games is also a great opportunity for recipients to show their appreciation of their donors' organs and the decisions made by the donors' families, with or without a donation will. Nevertheless, recipients often puzzle over how and what they should do for donor families: while some thank the families directly, others find themselves unable to speak to them.

3. Entrusting the Donor's Imaginary Life inside the Recipient's Body

Not all donor families attend the Transplant Games, but some use the opportunity to get to know recipients. When they have not met recipients, donor families can have very complex feelings and biased views toward them: some have very negative emotions such as jealousy, frustration, or even a kind of anger. After meeting and communicating with recipients, however, they often learn of recipients' appreciation of donors and donor families. They notice that although recipients and donor families are in different positions, they share the perception that the donor is the most important element in their lives. Donor families can come to entrust the donor's imaginary life to the recipient who received their transplanted living organs. One mother commented, "When I attended the Transplant Games I thought . . . it's all for the best: the best decision, the best thing for my son and our family. . . . To see from such a wide-ranging perspective how a human can save another human, it's just wonderful! When I see recipients I feel my son is valuable to others."

4. From Interdependent Relationships to Giving Their Love to the Donor's Life

Through the Transplant Games, donor families and recipients have discovered similarities in their situations, the most important being that both care strongly for donors' lives. Recipients need donors' organs to survive and donor families need recipients' bodies to keep their donors' organs alive. When both sides understand this, they can change dramatically in their attitudes to each other, moving to care about each other as a donor's organ senders and receiver. Many have found that they have constructed interdependent relationships, and they try to develop these to give their love to donors' lives through the same thoughts but different positions.

1. Transplant surgeons have been trying to calm tensions between recipients and donor families. Since the Japanese organ transplantation law prohibits meetings between recipients and donor families, some transplant surgeons attend the Transplant Games to support mutual understanding between the parties.
2. Recipients often want to see donor families to say thank you directly, but because of privacy protection issues they cannot have personal contact with them. Some recipients are also afraid to see donor families as they suspect that they will be blamed for being alive with the donors' organs after the families have suffered the loss of their loved ones. Most recipients find themselves in tears when they meet donor families at the Transplant Games and feel that they are charged by donor families with the mission of keeping the donors' organs alive with their own lives.
3. Most donor families feel isolated and depressed after organ donation and withdraw to the outskirts of society, regretting their donation decision. The Transplant Games serve as a catalyst to get to know each other and share the donor's life, helping them to construct an interdependent relationship with the recipients.

5. Interpreting the Donor's Life from Different Perspectives

The Transplant Games promote mutual understanding between recipients and donor families, and also serve to show that organ transplantation is a very complex and mysterious issue for humans. One transplant surgeon was so moved he could not speak when he saw recipients and donor families gathered the same place, sharing their feelings about donors. None of the participants had expected that such a day would be possible and he thought that perhaps the donor's life was present in each heart there. Recipients couldn't help crying—as a result of the Transplant Games they constructed partnerships with donor families and determined with them to live as long as possible to maintain the donor's life. Donor families recognize that recipients need donors' organs and that donor families need recipients' bodies to live, giving them a shared desire and purpose. The most important person to both is the donor; the most precious thing is the donor's life.

CREATING INTERRELATIONSHIPS: MOVING FROM ANTAGONISM TO MUTUAL UNDERSTANDING

This chapter introduced three schemes to boost mutual understanding between recipients and donor families—speaking out, thank you letters, and the Transplant Games.

1. Speaking out: recipients wanted to show their appreciation for organ donation to donor families but didn't know what to do for the donor family to show their appreciation. They were also wary of donor families' reactions, but interested to hear their feelings toward recipients. Simultaneously, donor families wanted to tell recipients about their experiences and feelings, and wanted to hear recipients' views.

2. Thank you letters: Japanese organ transplantation law prohibits recipients and donor families keeping in touch except through a thank you letter via JOTN, but most recipients did not write the letter because they had no idea what to say, and while some donor families eagerly awaited a letter, others did not expect or want one.

3. Transplant Games: the Japan Transplant Recipients Organization and transplant surgeons set up the games to encourage recipients' health development (figure 5.1). They also invited donor families to give recipients and donor families opportunities to meet and try to develop mutual understanding. As a result, all concerned parties began to construct interdependent relationships and to share their donors' imagined lives continuing.

The three categories of concerned party (transplant surgeons, recipients, and donor families) are very different and have various ways of

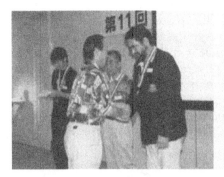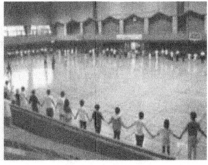

Figure 5.1.   Left: A donor father gives a recipient winner his award. Right: All the participants (transplant surgeons, recipients, and donor families) form a large "new life" circle, holding hands and sharing their various feelings toward the donors (Japan Organ Transplant Network, 2014). From www.jtr.ne.jp/japan_s/2002/sp11_photo.html.

understanding the situation surrounding organ transplantation, but nevertheless share mutual feelings of valuing donors. The speaking out activities were instigated by volunteers among both recipients and donor families. The concerns on either side concerning thank you letters also arose from their complex feelings based on sympathetic emotions toward each other. The tears welling up in many eyes at the Transplant Games resulted from their bitter experiences of the organ transplantation world that no one knew about before. But the buds of interrelationships among concerned parties are definitely appearing in various ways: slowly but steadily they are spreading, as despite their different perspectives and complex feelings they realize their mutual love and respect for donors and set out on the road to mutual understanding. The concerned parties' choice to start to build bridges between the different perspectives was a positive one and has only just begun.

NOTE

1. Additional data from the 23rd Japan Organ Transplant Games in Ishikawa (September 11–16, 2014): during the games and the week-long staff preparation, I gained useful new data and succeeded in completing follow-up research, adding updated or new information to the book.

REFERENCES

Fox, R., and Swazey, J. (1992). *Spare Parts: Organ Replacement in American Society*. New York: Oxford University Press.

Yasuoka, M. K. (2006). "Rebirthable Life: Medical Anthropology Study of the Concept of Life According to Concerned Parties Involved in Brain Death and Organ Transplantation." PhD thesis: Department of History and Anthropology (Medical Anthropology), Graduate School of Letters, Hokkaido University, Sapporo, Japan (unpublished).

———. (2010). "Medical Refugees in Japan: From Overseas Transplants to Organ Self-Sufficiency for Japanese Recipients." *Applied Ethics: Challenges for the 21st Century*. Sapporo, Japan: Center for Applied Ethics and Philosophy, Hokkaido University, 85–97.

———. (2013). "Rebirthable Life: Narratives and Reproductive Life of Japanese Brain-Dead Donors." *Research Journal of Graduate Students of Letters* (Japan) 8, 73–81.

SIX

Transforming Concepts of Life

INTRODUCTION

Cutting-edge medical technologies not only provide effective medical treatments but also create unforeseen issues for human beings. In particular, organ transplantation relies on new agents—donors—and their donated organs to save severely ill patients. Concerned parties—transplant surgeons, recipients, and donor families—have to deal with matters of life and death (including most frequently the donor's death, whether heart death or brain death; the organ donation; and the donor family's grieving process) whether they are prepared or not. Such an ambiguous human death, as a result of which partial organs are still alive although the whole body has legally died, has had unforeseen consequences for transforming concerned parties' concepts of life in various unpredictable ways. They find that they have to face and struggle with matters concerning the very nature of life (Namihira 1996).

The concept of organ transplantation is itself very simple and just involves transferring an organ from a dead person to a severely ill patient. Nevertheless, the pioneers of the treatment overcame great difficulties in finalizing the process and making it available to patients. According to the Hippocratic Oath sworn by physicians—"First, do no harm"— organ harvesting would appear to be against bioethics. Since this sensational medical treatment first started to save recipients, organ transplantation has been a magnet for gossip, rumors, and scandals. On the other hand, it has also shed light on aspects of altruistic and pure human love and created a new spirit of mutual assistance. Although everybody hopes that "no harm" will come to patients, the development of any cutting-edge medical treatment includes some risks to patients (Yasuoka 2006).

According to the narrative data collected from concerned parties, they feel (in various ways, depending on their relationship to the donor) that they produce "rebirthable life" from the donor's organ, which has a biologically limited life. Every concerned party naturally has a different perception of this "gift of life," and about the donor's existence in their own lives. Transplant surgeons experience changeable feelings toward recipients and donors (sometimes including donor families) and they are required to take into consideration both the recipient's and the donor's life when attempting to treat and save a patient. Recipients can consider that they gain "renewable life" from organ donation, but they feel resultant emotional burdens toward both donors and donor families. Donor families make the decision to donate an organ from a dead relative, but often feel that their family member's partial organs are still alive inside someone somewhere; thus, they have created an eternal life called "rebirthable life" for the donor in their imaginary world.

The new technology of organ donation has thus created three new ideas, with their own incipient issues, associated with changes in the concept of life.

1. The "gift of life": this catchphrase was created by British surgeon Dr. R. Calne and spread in the United States, stimulating America's feeling of humanity. However, in Japanese society, the custom of giving a seasonal gift requires the return of a reciprocal gift (usually of equal value). How and with what can recipients repay their organ donor?
2. "Renewable life": thanks to the development of organ transplantation, many recipients' failed organs have now become "renewable." Although recipients need donors to donate their organs, however, they are also very aware of the donor families who make the decision to donate. Transplant surgeons have to choose a moment to give up on saving a donor's life and focus on saving the recipient's body to make it renewable. Donor families, while grieving for the loss of their family member, can feel the continuation of the donor's organs in the renewed recipient's body through organ donation.
3. "Rebirthable life": most concerned parties spoke about the "rebirthable life" of the donor, a term used by one donor mother, but this is not the same as traditional beliefs in "rebirth." This is a unique and interesting phenomenon, which holds a measure of control over all concerned parties (Yasuoka 2013).

"GIFT OF LIFE": A DYSFUNCTIONAL RECIPROCITY

In Japan it is customary to exchange gifts twice a year with "Ochugen" (for a mid-year or summer gift) and "Oseibo" (for a year-end or winter gift). The system has two meanings: a superficial offer of greetings of the season, and an underlying hidden agenda that might be expressed as "I'll be counting on you in future." These two types of gift tend to be offered to someone who has done something for the giver, like a teacher or a boss. The senders also expect the receivers to offer a return gift, which is understood to involve a reciprocal effort or value. The return gifts are very varied: sometimes a material gift ranging from double to half the value of the original, and sometime a valuable effort on behalf of, or offer of support for, the sender. Recipients are under an obligation to senders and people are afraid to be considered ungrateful by others in Japanese society.

As a result of this Japanese traditional practice of exchanging gifts and the cultural obligations surrounding it, organ transplantation treatment has produced unusual dilemmas in Japan, giving rise to issues without parallel in other countries. In her work on organ transplantation, Fox and Swazey examined Marcel Mauss's "gift theory" and concluded that while all human societies have reciprocity systems to varying degrees, human organs in particular evoke "the tyranny of the gift" (Mauss 1954; Fox and Swazey 1992). In addition, Lock, who lived and undertook research in Japan, pointed out in her book that "[g]ift giving remains central to social solidarity in Japan. . . . This complex system of gift exchange requires an acute sensitivity to the obligations and the reciprocal worth embodied in a gift." She shows that organ donation in Japan is a much more difficult concept than it is in North American and European countries (Lock 2002). The narrative data of concerned parties to organ transplantation (transplant surgeons, recipients, and donor families) endorses the views of these sociologists and anthropologists, and the structure through which gift senders have power and recipients are controlled exists in varying degrees throughout the world.

All concerned parties spoke of the "gift of life" both positively and negatively: while assessing it as valuable, they also felt that it invited a dysfunctional reciprocity in practice. Some transplant surgeons, whose work included harvesting organs, were very negative toward the concept of the "gift of life," feeling instead that organ donation is a "gift of love" from donors to recipients. Others, who were more involved in transplanting organs into recipients, were very positive and mentioned how they felt the "gift of life" is a miraculous and dramatic medical treatment. Recipients frequently wondered what might be the most suitable gift in return for a donation of an organ and how to return such a gift to the donor or donor family, since the donated organ is not a material item but part of a human body. They felt they had a heavy load, carrying the expectations of the donor and donor family and the hope that they would survive, thus ensuring the survival of the dead person's organ. Donor families found themselves daily torn between satisfaction and regret as a result of their decision to donate their loved one's organ.

"GIFT OF LIFE" BY DONOR FAMILIES:
GIFTING THE DONOR'S THOUGHTS

The donor families are the final decision makers concerning organ donation, whether the donor has a donation will or not (after the revision of
the organ transplantation law family-presumed consent became available
if the donor had no donation will). According to my data, the most ideal
case of organ donation arises when a donor has an organ donation will;
however, in most cases this is not available and agreement to donate
relies on the bereaved families' decision. How do these people understand the "gift of life," who have had to choose to donate a dead family
member's organs? The narratives of donor fathers, mothers, and a wife
offer different assessments, reflecting their different relationships to the
donor.

1. Donor Father—Organ Donation of His Son with His Donation Will

Mr. Fukuzawa's son always talked about his donation will to other
family members, so the family consensus to donate his organ was easily
reached. The father was confident about the other family members'
agreement and explained that the organ donation following his son's
death, based on his donation will, was a very private matter for them.
Organ donation may be a "gift of life" for recipients but for these donor
family members, their priority was just to be true to the son's wish when
he was alive, and indeed the catchphrase "gift of life" evoked his son's
death and had negative connotations for this donor father.

2. Donor Father—Organ Donation of His Daughter without Her Donation Will

Mr. Sakamoto's daughter was killed suddenly in a car accident and
her doctor suggested organ donation, so the father and his family decided to go ahead, although she had no donation will. He did not use the
phrase of "gift of life" in his descriptions: he said that his doctor whispered, "There is a way to avoid your daughter's death through organ
donation." He agreed, thinking that this would bring his daughter eternal life. After the donation, however, he and his family were suspected of
receiving money from the hospital or a governmental organization. He
valued organ donation itself as a non-reciprocal gift because it comes
from donors and donor families whose spirits are full of sacrifice for
others. He expected nothing in return, but was eager to meet the recipient, feeling that this would enable him to meet his daughter inside the
recipient's body. He was too sad about losing his daughter to care about
the concept of the "gift of life."

3. Donor Mother—Organ Donation of Her Son with His Donation Will

Mrs. Fukuzawa knew about her son's donation will and didn't have any trouble or hesitation about agreeing to the donation. However, her grieving process was long and her recovery from her son's death very slow. Rather than her sorrow at losing her son diminishing, it grew deeper day by day. She said, "I agreed to my son's organ donation because he left his donation will: this is not a 'gift of life' for me, but just his wish. However, if he had not left a donation will, I couldn't have decided to donate. . . . Recently, I sometimes think that I would be against his organ donation, even if all my other family members agreed—I would still be strongly against it, alone."

4. Donor Mother—Organ Donation of Her Son without His Donation Will

Mrs. Noguchi's son had no donation will. He was an only child, and her husband was a patient in another hospital, so she had to decide on organ donation alone. Some medical staff put pressure on her to agree to donate, but it was the hardest decision of her life. She had no idea about organ donation and couldn't imagine whether her son had a donation will, as well as worrying about her husband's feelings. She couldn't say no to the medical staff so she agreed to the organ donation. When her son's body was back at home after the transplant, she felt she needed to apologize to him but she didn't know how. She lived in pain and sorrow until she received a thank you letter from a recipient: "I was only too happy to receive the letter and recognize that my son did a good deed." The thank you letter was the best reciprocal gift for her "gift of life."

5. Donor Mother—Organ Donation of Her Son with Her Own Donation Will

Mrs. Honda's son had no donation will when he had a car accident. She wanted to avoid his sudden death and offered her son's organs to his doctor for donation without consulting her husband and son (the donor's father and younger brother). She repeatedly said, "I didn't give a 'gift of life' at all: I didn't care about the recipients at that time, and I just thought about whether my son's organs, even partial organs, could live or not." She even stubbornly refused thank you letters and an award from the Ministry of Health, Labor, and Welfare in Japan, explaining that her organ donation decision was not for others or her nation, just for herself. She felt that she had not sent a "gift of life" because she felt her son was still alive, and thus she did not expect a return gift because she did not want to accept her son's death.

6. *Donor Wife—Organ Donation of Her Husband with His Donation Will*

Mrs. Suzuki knew of her husband's donation will and felt that achievement of his will was her mission as a wife (her husband has a donation will, she has a donation will of her husband, in addition, they discuss about organ donation issues before her husband suffered cancer). The "gift of life" and her husband's donation will happened to coincide, but she did not expect a reciprocal gift, although she would be happy to receive one because she would be happy to hear that her husband helped someone with his donation will. She said that she did not try to give a "gift of life," but that it is just the natural course of events to cycle from birth to death and back to life. She felt that donating her husband's organ was natural, and if she ever needs an organ transplant she will receive it as natural. She insisted that organ donation and reception are natural things for us as human beings, so nobody needs reciprocal gifts.

"GIFT OF LIFE" BY TRANSPLANT SURGEONS: RECEIVING THE DONOR'S WARM HEART

Transplant surgeons who receive a donor's love and transplant it via their organ into a recipient also have different understandings of the concept of the "gift of life."

1. *Heart Transplant Surgeon—"Gift of Love"*

Dr. Tanaka stated, "I don't like the term 'gift of life,' and some donor families don't like it either because organs are not material items, but 'gift' makes them sound like returnable objects." He continued, "It is a very rude expression for donors and donor families, I think: making the decision to donate organs is not easy, but I can't find a good alternative expression . . . although 'gift of love' is better than 'gift of life.'" He concluded that an organ donation cannot be taken back—it is just given to recipients by donors, and donors and donor families can't expect anything in return: they just give for the sake of severely ill patients. In essence, this surgeon did not originally want to perform organ transplant surgery because he was greatly shocked by the "Wada case" when he was a schoolboy. Instead, he wanted to be an artificial heart surgeon, but current medical treatment techniques are not yet advanced enough to support this career, so he uses organ transplant surgery to save patients as the very last option in their medical treatment.

2. *Heart Transplant Physician—"Slide of Life"*

Dr. Matsui said, "I think that organ donation and reception is a different quality of 'gift of life': giving someone life is a gift . . . but giving an organ is different from giving ordinary materials as gifts or presents. It doesn't mean that it passes from someone to someone else: we human beings are born and die repeatedly and we revert to earth after death and are reborn from earth again and again in a cycle. The same applies to our organs. I think, or I want to think, that this is a law of nature, so donor families don't have to think about giving organs to others and recipients don't feel so bad about being given organs from donors. In fact, donors are not giving their organs to recipients but just sliding organs from donors to recipients: that's it, I think." His understanding is that just as birth and death are natural parts of life, so organs should slide from one person to another naturally, as described by one of the fathers of liver transplantation, Dr. Starzl, in *The Puzzle People* (Starzl 1992). He continued, "I think that we should not think about organ donation as such a special thing and also recipients should not think so seriously about how to return such a gift."

3. Liver Transplant Surgeon — "Gift for Humans"

Dr. Aoki said proudly, "I believe that the people who know best about the wonder of organ transplantation are transplant surgeons, yes, we are, that why we can harvest organ and transplant organ, such a tough job! We know about the recipients who gained good health better than anyone, and I'm proud of that. It's why I appreciate the donors and donor families from the bottom of my heart." He analyzed the term "gift of life" and concluded that there are two meanings: having a severely ill patient come back to life through organ transplantation with donated organs and saving at least a part of the donor after their death. "The 'gift of life' is the ultimate gift for humans: we can't beat the gift of organ donation. So our great underlying gratitude for donors forms the basis of organ transplantation."

4. Kidney Transplant Surgeon (Eastern Japan) — "Gift of Patients"

Dr. Kawasaki lives in Tokyo in eastern Japan, where organ donation numbers are higher than in the more traditional western part of the country, although still very low compared with the rest of the world. He said, "I wonder whether the 'gift of life' refers not only to organ donation but also to the circumstances surrounding patients who are battling disease more widely. Of course, the narrowly defined meaning is 'organ donation,' but I think that we transplant surgeons have to pay attention to a much broader vision of helping patients." He insisted that organ transplantation in Japan is lagging significantly behind Europe and the United States as people focus on only the low organ donation numbers, the cultural barriers for recipients and surgeons' mistakes. While these reasons are broad and abstract, he recognized that gifts for patients also include overcoming their personal stresses and financial problems, as well as encouraging neighbors' positive opinions and communication, and creating socially permissive attitudes and environments.

5. Kidney Transplant Surgeon (Western Japan) — "Gift of Mutually Supporting Life"

Dr. Hasegawa lives in Osaka in western Japan, which is a more traditional region, making organ donation and reception more difficult than in eastern Japan. However, this surgeon also had a positive attitude to the term "gift of life." (My data show that transplant surgeons divide clearly into two types: one hesitates to use the term "gift of life" and the other admires it.) According to him, the phrase has two meanings: one for recipients and the other for donors. Recipients who are approaching death can live longer with donated organs, and the donors' organs can thus also live longer, even as partial transplants. These two incomplete bodies get together and one life survives longer. Donors' organs and recipients' bodies support each other and they live longer together, creating the wonderful "gift of life."

6. Kidney Transplant Surgeon (Veteran) — "Wonderful Human Gift"

Dr. Sasaki is one of the first generation of transplant surgeons in Japan (he was already at medical school at the time of the Wada case in 1968). He understood and accepted the unique tragic history of Japanese organ transplantation resulting from traditional culture combined with the Wada case and the subsequent mistrust of organ transplant treatment, leading to a long delay in its development in Japan compared with other countries. In addition, he had been battling against opponents in discussion of brain death and organ transplantation issues on TV programs and even took the witness stand in a courtroom. However, he gave a positive assessment of organ transplantation and admired it as the "gift of life," with the principle philosophy of donating organs for no rewards: wonderful evidence of humanity in the world.

"GIFT OF LIFE" BY RECIPIENTS: RETURNING A GIFT

The process of organ transplantation involves many concerned parties to create one "gift of life." It begins with donors' organ donations through donor families' decision making and continues with transplant surgeons' organ harvesting from donors and organ replacement into recipients' bodies. Only then can successful transplant surgery recipients recognize the "gift of life," but again their interpretations vary.

1. *"I Will Complete My Life to Be a Donor"*

Ai, who received an organ in Australia, always felt that, while she was very independent, she consulted her donor by asking her body before making any decisions and responding to its reaction before acting. (She said, "[W]ith my donor I am never by myself.") She felt that she combined herself with her donor in complete surrender, and her deep and sincere gratitude to the donor was autonomic. She decided that she would like to help someone after her death and wanted to donate her organs just as her donor did, completing her life as a donor. Her reciprocal gift is reliving her donor's experiences herself.

2. *"I Was Given Too Big a Gift Not to Reciprocate"*

Hana, who also received an organ in Australia, by contrast described her experience with a pessimistic voice and mood. Despite her negative attitude, she felt a deep sense of gratitude to her donor, but she was privately worried about receiving the "gift of life" and being unable easily to offer a reciprocal gift. Her experiences leading up to her organ reception were very convoluted, and complex emotions had preyed on her mind. In her case, organ transplantation, and especially the overseas transplant plan, was not her choice because she was still a child. She was too young to understand the "gift of life," or indeed conceive of what organ transplantation from a brain-dead donor involved. She grew up and married but admitted, "I can't even consult with my husband about my 'gift of life': it is too heavy an issue and too great a gift for me" as her eyes filled with tears.

3. *"I Will Live as Long as Possible in Return"*

Satoshi's was the second case of a simultaneous pancreas–kidney transplant from a brain-dead donor in Japan (his was the first case in eastern Japan). At that time, there were very few recipients from brain-dead donors, especially in Japan, so he was confused and puzzled about how to reciprocate to the "gift of life" givers (the donor and donor family) while maintaining confidentiality. However, his appreciation of his donor was so deep that he finally decided that he would try to live as long as he possibly can with the donor's organs, to please his donor and the donor family. He took great care of himself and kept in good health with the donated organ to try to keep it alive as long as possible, as his reciprocal gift for the "gift of life."

4. *"I Pray for Forgiveness from the Donor and Donor Family Every Night"*

Hiroshi responded to his American donor and donor family in two very different ways. He became the leader of one of the biggest recipient associations and worked hard as a volunteer with his colleagues; his activities were given a positive assessment by concern parties in the organ transplantation world. He also prayed quietly every night before sleeping and gave thanks for his donor, while begging forgiveness of both the donor and the donor family. His two kinds of reciprocal gift are diverse in content, but both convey his honest feelings toward his "gift of life" giver.

5. "I'm Taking the Lead in Promoting Organ Transplantation"

Akira is the leader of one of the country's organ recipient associations and spends most of his time outside work undertaking activities for the association. He took the lead in promoting organ transplantation in a very affirmative and positive way, and showed a calm and reassuring attitude in his advocating activities, while aiming to increase organ donation numbers. He claimed, "We organ recipients know best how wonderful treatment organ transplantation is. We should show these ourselves: first, by living longer with the donated organ; and second, by using our 'gift of life' [to] offer something in return for donors and donor families." He expects human life and society to improve through the altruism of organ donation, as appreciation builds for the sacrifice donors make for others, refusing to be indifferent to human relationships and ways of removing pain.

6. "I Will Tell People What It Is Like to Be Involved in Organ Transplantation"

Ken is a volunteer worker in one of the organ advocating parties. He felt that Japanese organ transplantation lagged far behind other countries, especially the United States. His response was, "First, we need education and second, information for Japanese people, because too many are not interested in organ transplantation." He tried to tell people what it is like to be involved in organ transplantation in his voluntary activities, which were his life's work, saying, "Organ transplantation is a wonderful medical treatment and I experienced the 'gift of life' that is organ reception. Organ transplantation is equal to the 'gift of life,' actually giving life and precious human love to others through altruism: I feel and know it through my experience. I think organ recipients really appreciate donors and donor families: that is why our mission should be to tell people about our wonderful experiences, educating children and giving information to adults about health promotion. When Japanese people learn the wonder of organ transplantation, this is my way of showing my appreciation as a reciprocal gift."

7. "I Try to Attend Any Donor Family Events"

Takeshi, who received organs from his mother as a living donor and more than ten years later a heart-dead donor in Japan, tried to attend any donor family gatherings he could to understand their feelings. With two donors, his appreciation for the "gift of life" was much stronger and more complex, although it was his second donation that stimulated his grateful feelings toward his first donor. At the same time, not only positive feelings of gratitude but also negative feelings of regret were evoked, so while his appreciation for the two donors was much stronger than before, he also experienced more complex feelings against the "gift of life." His gift in return for his luck at receiving two organ donations is to try to pass on the human love he received to others.

1. One response of recipients to the issue of reciprocation for the "gift of life" is to live as long as possible, meaning that the donor's precious organ is treasured, and showing the advantage of the donor family's decision to donate their loved one's organ. Most recipients spoke about living as long as possible and keeping the organ alive: some focused on the organ's life but others on the recipient's life with the donated organ.

2. A second response is for recipients to become involved in advocating activities concerning organ donation and transplantation within Japanese and international practices, both to support organ recipients and to encourage recipient candidates. Recipients know the anxieties about organ transplantation faced by recipient candidates, so they offer workshops themselves or attend transplant surgeons' study meetings. They also take part in combined social events with recipients and donor families to inform Japanese society about the effectiveness of organ transplantation.

3. A third response is for recipients to thank donors and donor families, including living donors. These recipients actively participate in efforts to build mutual understanding with donor families to learn about their feelings and emotional issues. However, although living donors are alive, cadaveric donors are gone forever, so recipients can only contact the bereaved donor families.

The next section introduces the new concept of "renewable life," investigating the various differences in perspectives related to the positions of concerned parties.

"RENEWABLE LIFE": REPLACING ORGANS
IN A BIOLOGICALLY LIMITED BODY

Organ transplantation is also called "organ replacement," through which a patient suffering from severe organ failure can receive a replacement functioning organ from a living or dead donor. This terminology can give the impression that the recipients have survived death and that their life has been renewed. Nevertheless, the replacement organ's second life is also biologically limited, and someday the recipient will die, as will the donated organ. In other words, organ replacement does not lead to eternal life; it simply postpones the recipient's biological death. In fact, this "renewable life" brings a double risk of death, as the recipient faces two potentially deadly risks: failure of the donated organ and rejection of the organ or other unexpected complications within the recipient's body. The basic philosophy of the "gift of life" may sound harmonious, but "renewable life" also has biological limitations for both the donor's organ and the recipient's life, although—thanks to the continuing development of medical technology—recipients now also have the option to try retransplantation if a replacement organ fails.

Many people believe that organ transplantation offers recipients the promise of the "gift of life" and a rosy future. Transplant surgeons know the limitations of an organ's life-span and the problems of organ rejection, despite immunosuppressant therapy. Nevertheless, although organ transplantation has many obstacles, it is often the only way save a severely ill patient. Recipient candidates learn about side-effects and other troublesome symptoms from their doctors but may fail to grasp the medical advice and information in full because they are only amateurs, not medical experts. Donor families are just bereaved families of people who have died suddenly and often unexpectedly, and thus often have access to even less information about the organ transplantation process and its potential outcomes. Organ replacement thus starts with very unequal levels of knowledge and communication among concerned parties.

"RENEWABLE LIFE" BY TRANSPLANT SURGEONS:
DILEMMAS AND MISSIONS

Transplant surgeons provide "renewable life" for their severely ill patients. How do they understand and describe this new concept of life, given their different perspectives on their roles?

1. "Should I Save a Donor First?"

Dr. Tanaka explained disconsolately, "Whenever I harvest a heart from a brain-dead donor to save a recipient I always think that I should try harder to save the donor first. We doctors can't help trying to save a dying person whenever he/she is in front of us: that is our job! Don't you agree? That is our reaction as a human being, too, right? We are only human as well as being doctors! A recipient can live biologically without the new heart's function, and a donor's heart is alive biologically without the body's brain. I wonder whether both the recipient and donor are still partially alive and partially dead." He reflected on the conundrum of what biological life in fact entails: does the "renewable life" of recipients need a "non-renewable life" from donors?

2. "One Death Is Better than Two!"

Dr. Matsui said, "One death is better than two!" without any hesitation. According to him, if it is possible to save a brain-dead patient, of course that takes priority, but it is still impossible for brain-dead patients to survive with current medical techniques. In addition, a beating heart from a brain-dead donor is a requirement of a heart transplant to keep a severely ill patient alive, because alternatives such as artificial organs, xenotransplantation (using animal organs), regenerated organs, and induced pluripotent stem cells (iPS) are still at the experimental stage. He insisted that a doctor's mission is to save even one life to make it "renewable" rather than none, if at all possible.

3. "A Little Love from Donors Saves Recipients"

Dr. Aoki described his dissatisfaction with the present situation in Japan, which has the worst levels of organ shortages in the world. (Although the number of organ donations from brain-dead donors rose after the revision of the organ transplantation law, Japan still has the severest organ shortage in the world.) "We know very well that we can't save either heart-dead or brain-dead donors' lives yet, unfortunately. And we also know that we can save recipients' biological lives through organ replacement, fortunately, but we have to depend on organ donations. The present state of our medical service is not enough, but a little love from donors and donor families via organ donation can save patients with severe organ failure. Although we can't save both lives, one life and a partial organ can be saved through organ transplantation."

4. "Organ Replacement Makes the Recipient's Life Renewable"

Dr. Kawasaki spoke excitedly about how organ transplantation is a wonderful medical treatment for patients and a miracle phenomenon for the world of science. "It was once considered impossible that another's organ could enter a body and the transplanted organ engraft successfully. This is an abnormal condition except in pregnancy. . . . From a scientific point of view transplant surgeons are endlessly interested in organ replacement as a way to renew human life biologically: it is very challenging research but worthwhile work for the results."

5. *"Non-Renewable Dead People Save Renewable Patients"*

Dr. Hasegawa insisted, "There are various assessments of organ transplantation but I think that it is a superb medical service for both recipients and donors, because recipients can renew their organs and live longer, while donors can live on, even though only through partial organs. Both biological lives are made longer though organ replacement. I cannot think of a reason not to perform organ transplantation; however, I'm not happy yet because we still cannot cure recipients' failed organs and we still cannot help donors' bodies, except the donated organs."

6. *"Donors Can Renew Recipients' Organs"*

Dr. Sasaki said, "Organ transplantation is a wonderful treatment, I think, because thanks to organ donation recipients' failed organs can be renewed. Donors cannot live anymore, but some of their partial organs are still functioning biologically, and can be donated to support recipients. When people leave this world for heaven, they can say, 'Please use my organs for severely ill patients who need an organ transplant.' Donors' human love, medical technology and surgeons' skills combine and patients can renew their lives. I believe that organ transplantation is a miracle in the human world."

"RENEWABLE LIFE" BY RECIPIENTS: GRATITUDE AND GUILT

Recipients whose lives have been renewed by donors' organs described their rational understanding of the process of organ replacement.

1. *"I'm Sharing My Renewed Life with My Donor's Liver"*

Ai explained, "If I had not received a donated liver at that time in Australia, I would surely have died about ten years ago. After the organ replacement I felt sure that my donor was male, although he is now in my female body. Actually I can feel him: I feel his liver here." (She held my hand to her stomach.) "My liver was replaced with the donor's organ and my life was saved. My donor passed away and I am alive now. However, a partial piece of his body—that is, his liver—is still alive and functioning in my body now. I'm sharing my renewed life with my donor's liver. His liver and my body without the liver were put together and produced renewed life. Every morning starts with him so I speak to him, saying, 'Good morning, you are fine today too!'"

2. "I've Accepted My Donor's Remaining Time"

Hana said, "I received my liver from a brain-dead donor but I understand that he gave me his time. If he hadn't had a car accident, he should have lived longer—until eighty years old, maybe. He died suddenly, leaving his remaining life time. . . . He gave me a huge gift." She felt that she renewed the donor's liver: his functioning liver replaced her failed one and she is alive now having succeeded, via his liver, to the rest [of] the time that would have been allocated [for] his life. She felt that two biologically limited lives joined in her body and created a new gift of "renewable life," but which was also a limited life. She claimed, "I had to live two lives: it is so tough for me to live this renewed life. I appreciate my donor but it is too heavy a 'gift of life' when I think about this issue."

3. "I Try to Improve the Shelf Life of My Renewed Organs"

Satoshi said that he would not be alive now without his organ donations, so he was trying to improve and extend the life of his renewed organs because they gave him life. His donor died and his original organs had failed, but the donor's biologically living organs began functioning or living in his body. He felt that by his body living longer with the renewed organs, he was extending not only his life but also the life of the donor's partial organs.

4. "I'm Using My Renewed Life for the Good of Others"

Hiroshi explained, "I think that I was selected to be an organ recipient; it sounds awfully arrogant, though. But there are many recipient candidates waiting for organ donations, so why me? I appreciate my donor and the donor family, of course, but I was extremely lucky, so I also thank God. That's why I have a duty to use my biologically renewed body for the good of others as my mission. I was given the 'gift of life' but I strongly feel that I was chosen and given 'luck' by God. Although I can't understand God's meaning, he sent me a renewed life, so I'm doing what I imagine he wants of me. I sometime feel that I am alive through God or through luck from God, so I feel my mission to work for others strongly."

5. "I Want to Recommend Organ Transplantation for Other Patients"

Ken stated, "I think organ transplantation is the most wonderful thing but only a few people know about this amazing treatment and most are not interested in organ transplantation. I was so happy that I could accept an organ transplant, because I had very tough days during dialysis: dialysis treatment wasn't a match for my body so I became depressed and I really prepared for my own death. After the donor's organ was replaced in my body I was renewed, not only in my kidney but also my character, and I became a person with a sunny disposition. I feel that everything is great for me now, so I want to tell others (especially recipient candidates) all about organ transplantation. There are many people who don't even know that organ donation from living spouses is possible now."

6. "I'm Following the Path I Believe in with My Renewed Life"

Akira said, "I was struggling with my life during dialysis because I couldn't work and I have sons of school age: I thought I couldn't die before they were at least twenty years old. Fortunately, I received a kidney from [a] brain-dead donor in Japan and I'm working ten hours per day with my renewed body. I can't thank my donor enough, and I don't know how to repay my gratitude to the donor family. I understand their feelings when they frown to see recipients, because we renewed our bodies with the donor's organs but the donors died. So I'm following the path I believe in with my renewed life."

7. "I'd Like to Spend Most of My Re-Renewed Time Helping Others"

Takeshi said, "I was so lucky to receive organs twice in my life: receiving an organ donation even once in a lifetime is a very lucky situation because of the severe organ shortage. My first renewed kidney failed soon because I did not care enough for myself, but despite my carelessness I had the great chance of a second organ donation. I had my heart set on spending most of my re-renewed time helping others strongly and I've been trying every day, but not enough." According to his narrative, he regretted his first renewed life and he spends his time undertaking activities of human love, helping others. However, he never touched on the topic of his donor family, and he excused himself from it, saying, "I can't understand their feelings, and I can't say anything for them, just show appreciation: that's all!"

"RENEWABLE LIFE" BY DONOR FAMILIES: DONOR FAMILIES AND DONORS

Organ replacement and biologically "renewable life" are only for organ recipients, not for donors. While the donors support the "renewable life" of recipients, they themselves die, except via their partial donated organs. After their "gift of life" of organ harvesting for recipients, donors' lives are over and their families are bereaved. However, their partial organs continue to function inside the recipients' bodies and produce "renewable life" and their bereaved families become donor families.

1. "I'm Proud of My Son's Donation Will to Renew Someone"

Mr. Fukuzawa donated his son's organ with his donation will. According to his narrative, in cases where the donor's donation will is clear, donor families tend to separate the events surrounding the organ donation from the issues concerning the donor's death. He said, "I'm proud of my son's donation will to renew someone. We knew his will very well and what he was like, and knew he must be happy to hear about his organs being donated and that he renewed other people in this world. All his family members can vouch for his satisfaction. To be honest, my son's death . . . I can't believe that my son's life is over—he was such a special son—he can't renew his life, but he renewed other people. . . . That's why my son is a special person, his sacrificing spirit and behavior of organ donation is still alive in someone's body brilliantly."

2. "I Want to See the Recipient Who Keeps My Daughter in Her Renewed Body"

Mr. Sakamoto, who donated his daughter's organ without a donation will, felt a mixture of sadness for his lost daughter and deeply apologetic feelings for his decision to donate her organs without her permission. This caused him strong emotional issues for a long time. He whispered, "If I could—it is impossible, I know—but if I could, I want to see the recipient who received my daughter's kidney. I would like to touch her stomach where my daughter's kidney replaced and I want to ask my daughter in the recipient's renewed body, 'Was my decision to donate your organ good? Do you forgive your dad?'" He continued, crying: "The donor might respond to me, but I really want to hear my daughter's answer. That's my dream: that my daughter is in a recipient's renewed body and she is alive somewhere as a missing child."

3. "Renewing Two Lives through Organ Donation"

Mrs. Honda donated her son's organ without his donation will: she offered organ donation to her son's doctor when she knew he had no hope for survival after a car accident. She thought about it over and over again and remembered a TV program about a donor who had a "renewable life" and she thought that this is a great idea to keep her son live even if only kidneys in someone's body (two kidney recipients). She decided, "This is the only way to keep my son alive: even a partial organ can keep his biological life going." According to her narrative, she decided to donate her son's organ to keep its biological life alive in the recipient's body, meaning that the recipient also got a "renewable life" as a result.

4. "Whether Recipients' Lives are Renewed or Not, I'm Sad about My Son's Death"

Mrs. Fukuzawa, who donated her son's organs with his donation will, found that the organ donation and her son's death were completely different events for her at that time. She recounted disconsolately, "Death, the death of my son is so sad and people can't know how others feel until they are in our shoes." While she was happy that her son's organ donation gave some people "renewable life," her son's organ donation and his death were not connected for her, and she said, "Whether recipients' lives are renewed or not, I'm sad about my son's death more than anything else." Her son donated in Australia but if he had donated in Japan and if she had the opportunity to see the renewed recipient, she felt that she would have had the chance to reduce her sadness.

5. "If My Son Helped Renew Someone's Life, I'm Happy"

Mrs. Noguchi donated her son's organs without his donation will, and wept bitterly. She reported that she sometimes felt jealous about recipients' renewable lives and smiled sadly at the bitter memories. However, she quickly found that her mind changed when she had an opportunity to meet recipients, and she said, "I was so happy to see recipients who looked healthy and I strongly feel that my son helped others. Organ replacement makes a severely ill patient's body renewable and my son contributed, so that's wonderful, isn't it?"

6. "My Husband Died and Someone Received 'Renewable Life' Naturally"

Mrs. Suzuki donated her husband's organs with his donation will, and felt that organ donation itself helped to heal her grief. He was a brain surgeon during his life, so his organ donation had a special meaning, and she did it as her wifely mission. Because he had studied and taken care of patients for many years, his dream was that organ replacement should create "renewable life" for recipients. Although he passed away, his wife made his dream come true through her love for her husband. Now, whenever she meets renewed recipients, it makes her so happy, even though she was so sad about losing her husband. Nevertheless, she wondered how she would react in different circumstances, saying, "I can't have the same feelings toward my daughter. There are different feelings between my children and my spouse. I might instead be jealous to see a renewed child with my child donor's organ!"

1. Transplant surgeons' assessments of organ transplantation and "renewable life" are extremely positive because both "renewable life" and "rebirthable life" are considered forms of survival by medical staff—both are wonderful. They are satisfied that their

organ replacement techniques can provide "renewable life" for severely ill patients. The technology also stimulates their curiosity as scientists.

2. Organ recipients also rate organ transplantation and "renewable life" highly, but they cannot simply be pleased, and have complex feelings, combining happiness and guilt. They fear being judged by donor families and feel frustration at not being appreciated. They struggle to seek their own rationalization for spending their daily life with renewed biological bodies containing donors' partial functioning organs. Some recipients feel they share their renewed lives with their donors, while others feel that they have received new lives and try to contribute to social activities for others. Their interpretations of "renewable life" are various and unpredictable, but they feel strong appreciation for the development of medical technology, transplant surgeons' techniques, donors' organ donations, and their families' decisions.

3. Donor families either love or hate the idea of "renewable life." They understand that organ donation is for organ replacement, which produces "renewable life." Their positive outlook is that a patient received a renewable body thanks to the donor's noble organ donation, so they can feel proud of their family member. Their more negative assessment is that the partial organs giving "renewable life" are the donor's, and they dislike the implication that the donor's precious organs are just perceived as replaceable material items.

The next section describes the new concept of the continuing life of donors among concerned parties (transplant surgeons, recipients, and donor families) in Japan. It traces their unique history as they have alternated between hope and fear, and between joy and grief toward donors—the new agent in the emerging medical technology of organ transplantation.

"REBIRTHABLE LIFE": FROM ORGAN TO WHOLE BODY WITH ETERNAL LIFE

Organ transplantation is called the "gift of life," but organ donation itself is not a gift that gives life because the organ alone is not a material item and nobody can present life itself like a Christmas present. The real practice of organ transplantation is organ replacement: recipients receive a replacement for their failed organ and feel that their body is renewed with donated organs from a donor's donation will. Donor families experience various changing emotional interpretations of donating the organs of their family members (most often their children), yet at heart they are just bereaved families. If organ donation is called the "gift of life" and recipients renew their failed organs, how should the donor's life be recognized by concerned parties in reality?

Transplant surgeons know both organ givers (donors and donor families) and takers (recipients) and they explain that both the harvesting and the transplantation of organs are dramatic events. They feel that they become mediators between the donor and recipient, and emotionally that they support the giving and receiving of human love from donor and donor family to recipients. Recipients feel the donors' organs inside their bodies, and may even believe that they feel their donors as invisible presences, and as evidence of the continuing existence of the donors via their organs (according to my interview data from 2002). However, transplant medical treatment has, of course, been developing over the last several years. Organs can now be preserved much longer inside brain-dead bodies before transplant. Transplanted organs now also work much longer than before; thus, transplant surgeons have to refuse organ transplantation to recipients who are too severely ill if there is no hope of their surviving very long, giving priority to patients whose lives may be extended by more than a year with the transplant. This refusal of the operation is another new tough job for transplant surgeons (according to my follow-up research data from 2014).

Transplant surgeons can touch the donors' organs and recipients can feel the organs inside their bodies, but donor families cannot see the donors after their death. Despite saying goodbye to their loved ones at cultural death rituals such as funerals, cremations, burials, and other mourning events, they cannot fully accept the donors' deaths because the donors' partial organs are functioning inside other bodies. Recipients appreciate organ donation and are happy to receive "renewable life," but donor families can't expect the same. They have to try to recognize that organ donation is a wonderful thing and that the donors' partial organs are supporting the recipients while simultaneously experiencing the loss of a family member. Thus, the concept of donors' "rebirthable life" was created.

"REBIRTHABLE LIFE" BY TRANSPLANT SURGEONS

All concerned parties—transplant surgeons, recipients, and donor families—have special feelings toward donors that are difficult to explain rationally but reflect their different positions.

1. "Harvesting the Donor's Love"

Compared with other organ transplant surgeons, Dr. Tanaka's description of the process was the most shocking. One reason for this is that he had to harvest still-beating organs from donors; another is that in all countries the symbol of the heart is used as a metaphorical representation, with several meanings outside its blood-pumping organic function. This heart transplant surgeon insisted that, "It should be 'gift of LOVE' not 'gift of life' because donors are only thinking of someone else's life and health. . . . We receive donated organs, so I hardly dare to say something about donors and donor families. . . . I transplant donors' organs into recipients who can take care of the organ and the donor families' feelings." He understood that donors can gain "rebirthable life" invisibly and eternally in an imaginary world among donor families.

2. "Great Dramatic Life"

Dr. Matsui's assessment of organ transplantation was of a "great dramatic life" for both recipients and donors (including donor families). He had witnessed a lot of dramatic episodes that showed him transplantation's basis in human love. He complained about the worldwide issues surrounding organ transplantation and insisted that the job is a very tough one, involving routine medical treatments twenty-four hours a day, every day of the year. Most heart transplants depend on overseas donors so he had to fly abroad with recipient candidates; he continued to communicate with patients and families in the United States. In spite of such a tough job, he could see and feel the impressive and beautiful human drama created through organ donation and replacement and by donor families giving donors a second life.

3. "We Should Be Aware of the Treasure of the Donor's Life"

Liver transplants depend on either brain-dead donors or living donors, whose risks are also high. Dr. Aoki insisted on the wonder of organ transplantation but also stressed the importance of organ donation, saying, "We should be aware of the treasure of the donor's life." What he meant by this was not animated life like that of recipients or donor families but something that included the organs themselves, the donation will, the organ donation, and the donor family's decision to donate the organs. He found meaning in donors' lives because their organs continue to function inside the recipients, as "a treasure in this world." Donors' lives also offer "rebirthable life" so that this transplant surgeon can save recipients' lives and offer encouragement to donor families because the donors' partial organs are still functioning both for recipients and donor families.

4. "Supernatural Power of the Donor's Life"

Dr. Kawasaki's impression of the donor's life was created for him when he was a medical student and decided to be a transplant surgeon.

He listed many reasons that organ transplantation is a wonderful thing, such as the development of medical technology, surgeons' skills, recipients' perseverance over physical pain and mental difficulties, and donor families' decisions to donate organs. However, he felt that organ donation was such a wonderful and mysterious matter beyond human understanding that it actually had a supernatural power, creating invisible and eternal "rebirthable life." He said, "Organ donation is a part of the 'gift of life' and a way each one of the members of the human race can individually help each other. I think that the concept of the 'gift of life' can spread wider meanings in human society. One of the practical ways to do this is through organ donation. It makes a vivid impression on us!"

5. *"We Can Save the Donor's Life Partially"*

Dr. Hasegawa's assessment of the donor's life was very rational and unusual in the Far East. His statement was very objective and pointed out that organ transplantation is a very thorny medical issue with many troubling aspects, but that transplant surgeons have to maintain a cool demeanor to perform their crucial role. The fact is that the donor is dead by law, but the donor's organs are still biologically functioning for a short time after "official" human death, although not indefinitely. Organ harvesting takes advantage of the time lag before the organs' biological death. As a result, recipients can survive with donors' organs, which continue to function inside recipients, meaning that surgeons can save the donor's life partially, creating "rebirthable life" for the organs.

6. *"Enchanting Donor's Life"*

Dr. Sasaki's understanding of the donor's life was very philosophical, perhaps as a result of his longevity: he was aware of the history of organ transplantation in Japan—both its positive and negative aspects. His narrative outlined both cool rationalism and heartwarming episodes, as his experiences covered both the bright and dark sides of organ transplantation. He said, "Organ transplantation is wonderful, especially . . . as it has produced 'an enchanting donor's life' or 'rebirthable life' for recipients. Without organ transplantation we would have no 'gift of life' and no 'donor's life' either. I feel the donors' lives: they tell us a great deal about what human love is and indeed what life is. We can learn a lot from the donor's life, which is such a beautiful and mysterious existence for us." He stated that for transplant surgeons the donor's "enchanting" or "rebirthable" life reduced the dilemma and the guilt of organ transplantation, allow them to reduce their guilt toward the donor families.

"REBIRTHABLE LIFE" BY RECIPIENTS

How do the recipients who had donor's organs transplanted feel about the "rebirthable life" of donors?

1. "I Have Taken to Consulting My Donor When I Make a Decision"

Ai felt that her (male) donor's liver was living inside her and that she was sharing her life with the donor: she created a subservient relationship with her donor. She was very close to death in an Australian hospital when she was waiting for an organ, and was lucky to receive one and be able to live an ordinary life again. She really appreciated her donor, and felt her donor's human love strongly. "There is true love in organ donation because donors don't expect any reward at all. I couldn't live without my donor, so I obey him in everything. If I have a dilemma I have taken to consulting my donor when I make a decision . . . and I obey his opinion." Her donor became her life partner and she constructed an idea of the donor's life inside her, sharing her renewed body.

2. "I Try Not to Think about My Donor"

Hana had a negative interpretation of organ transplantation. A large factor in this experience was that she was a girl when she received the organ and her doctor and parents decided on the transplant but it was not her choice. When she grew up, therefore, she faced the problem of accepting her position as a recipient. "I try not to think about my donor. I appreciate my donor and I recognize that I received a big thing from my donor, but it is too difficult and painful to think about it: it is too tough an issue for me." She broke off, weeping. Later, she said, "He had some time until his natural death, but he died early as a result of a car accident, and I received the rest of his time. I accepted it, this 'rebirthable life' of his, and I am keeping it instead of him." She apologized but said, "Can I stop thinking about my donor?" We can learn much from her narration about the greater issues and difficulties surrounding children's organ reception and the existence of donors for them.

3. "I Feel There Is Nothing More Precious in This World than Donors"

Satoshi's narration was very positive and he was full of appreciation for his donor and trying to keep the donor's organs safely inside his body for as long as possible. His attitude to his donor's life was detached from his donor's existence and he did not feel that he shared his life with his donor's. However, he struggled to find a way to show his gratitude to his donor, the donor's family members, all his medical staff (especially the transplant surgeons), and his parents. He was a modest and quiet person so he did not show great emotion, but he insisted, "I think that donors' organ donation is the most precious human love and behavior toward others in this world." His interpretation of his donor's "rebirthable life" was that he should live as long as possible for his donor in return. In typical traditional Japanese male style he tried to show his appreciation through his behavior rather than words.

4. *"I Nearly Had Signed Off but I Once More Woke from Death by My Donor"*

Hiroshi told a unique tale about his donor's life. "I have to hide my face from my donor family, so I can only say thank you in my prayers, but I often feel that I was selected as his/her recipient and I was made alive by my donor to do something to help others. I can't understand or find the reason why I should receive an organ and survive except through my donor's will, and he/she gave me a mission." He also cared about whether his donor and the donor family would forgive him from the bottom of his heart: his donor had died and the donor family grieved but he alone was happy to receive the organ and survive. "Thanks to organ donation recipients can live but donor families have no such good results." While he accepted the donor's "rebirthable life," he could only feel it emotionally and "virtually," but he wanted to grasp it with his hands and touch the donor as if they were a living being.

5. *"Everyone Should be a Donor"*

Ken's interpretation of his donor's life was also positive. He said, "I became a very positive person after the organ transplant and I became active too. . . . I have received an organ from my donor so I have to tell others how both organ reception and donation are wonderful and how we are so grateful to donors and donor families for making us recipients happy. I think that everyone should donate organs and become a donor." He had opportunities to discuss organ transplant issues at home with his wife and sons, but was hesitant about touching on his donor and when talking about his donor's life, became silent. It seems that the relationship between recipients and their donors' lives is very sensitive and delicate: it causes dilemmas and their feelings change day by day.

6. *"I Would Like to Share My Feelings for My Donor with Donor Families"*

This kidney recipient's interpretation of organ transplantation was neutral and objective. He was aware that all concerned parties hold different opinions and place different values on the concept of life. He understood that, while there is no initial connection, after organ transplantation a new bond is formed between donor families and recipients, with donors at its center, meaning that donor families and recipients have started creating and developing new relationships, centered on donors. "I have no idea what we should do. And what do donor families expect us to do for them? I'm feeling my way myself, and I can only try to imagine what donor families may expect from us recipients." His description showed that recipients have no words or actions to express their thanks directly to donors for their lives.

7. "I've Become a Different Person since I Was Given Another Organ"

Takeshi's attitude toward two donors was interesting: he recounted that the relationship between donors and recipients was changeable. His first donor was a living donor and his second a cadaveric donor, for whom he can create the donor's life in his imaginary world. "I've become a different person since I was given another organ," he said. He had not changed after the first donation, but changed absolutely after the second. The difference did not arise from whether the organ came from a living or a cadaveric donor, but from a first organ transplant and a retransplantation. He feels that donors love the second organ transplant recipient even more than the first one: "Even one organ donation is lucky, but retransplant recipients are twice as lucky, so I also have twice as great a responsibility. I'm trying to take care of other recipients to show my double appreciation for donors and donor families."

"REBIRTHABLE LIFE" BY DONOR FAMILIES

Organ transplantation has produced new agents: from deceased patients and bereaved family it has created donors and donor families. However, although in Japan people pay attention to donors and recipients, the donors' bereaved families sometimes get forgotten and their grief at losing a family member (often a child) can be glossed over. They ask to be referred to as "donor families" rather than bereaved families because they feel that the donors are still alive in their imaginary world through their "rebirthable life" in the recipient's body. The donor family feels that the donor's life is still close to them.

1. "My Son Gives Me a Supportive Push"

Mr. Fukuzawa donated his son's organ with a donation will, but despite the family's consensus on the donation, their sadness as a bereaved family was very deep and his wife was sick in bed for a while. He could not discuss his son's death, but felt that his son was present in his mind. He described his feelings: "My son gives me a supportive push in my back, since his 'rebirthable life' so I can work on activities for the donor family club. He says, 'I died and donated my organs for severely ill patients as your son, so cheer up and you should work for someone else in trouble like me, Dad!'" His son was reborn in his mind and provided advice to his father, helping him maintain a constructive father/son relationship as if he were still alive. As a result of this invisible relationship the donor was reborn in the world of his imagination.

2. "My Daughter Became a Missing Child Somewhere in Japan"

Mr. Sakamoto donated his daughter's organ with no donation will, and the family reached consensus on the donation without a problem. Although there was family consent, however, he was emotionally scarred by other relatives and his neighbors, as they accused him of having received money in exchange for his daughter's organs, and of causing her body pain after death from the organ harvest. This led him to wonder whether his daughter resented her father for donating her organ without her permission or whether she was happy to donate and help a lady recipient. He strongly wanted to speak with his daughter heart to heart, but could only manage an impersonal one-way communication. However, he joined in with donor families' activities and tried to meet recipients directly at various events. His daughter was reborn in his mind and he felt that she was whispering voicelessly into his heart through her "rebirthable life." He felt her presence, not as reborn into the family house, but as if she was still present in the world but had become missing, or had even left home to get married and live elsewhere.

3. "My Son Is with Me All the Time"

Mrs. Honda donated her son's organ with neither a donation will nor family consensus, because when he died she and her husband were almost divorced and her younger son was too young to discuss his older brother's organ donation. After the donation, she left western Japan for northern Japan with her younger son, and lived in a small apartment with no neighbors. She felt that her son was always with her: "I lived with my sons at that time in an unknown place: my older son was with me all the time and my younger son was too little to leave alone." Outside her home she pretended to be a single mother with an only son, but at home she was the mother of two boys. "We had a funeral for him, where I pretended to be a bereaved mother who had lost her son but I knew I had kept him alive through the donation. I celebrated my older son's birthday with my second boy at home." This donor mother donated her son's organ to avoid his death, and felt that he was reborn. She and her younger son made a new family in their new home in new town, and the donor's "rebirthable life" was created.

4. "That's the Sort of Generous Person He Was"

Mrs. Fukuzawa also donated her son's organ with a donation will. Family members knew his will so it was not difficult for them to agree to organ donation, and their friends and neighbors understood this attitude and admired his decision, saying, "Organ donation? That's the sort of generous person your son was: always trying to help others!" However, her grief was very deep and long, reaching a serious level of dysfunctionality and lasting more than ten years. Her husband tried not to mention their son's death, although in fact she accepted it and created her son's memory in her mind very clearly as a "rebirthable life." Although she understood her son's death and greatly admired his donation will, she felt that he would never be reborn like before his brain death, and only his partial organs were alive somewhere. This made her very confused.

5. "I Feel My Son Whenever I Meet Recipients"

Mrs. Noguchi donated her son's organ without a donation will and after she had already lost all her other family members. In addition, when she saw her son's body after the organ donation she thought that his face had changed: she had a great shock and felt regret for a long time. However, when she had a chance to meet surviving organ recipients, she felt her son's existence: "I feel my son whenever I meet recipients. I don't know who has my son's organs and I don't know where they are. But my son's donated organs are surely alive somewhere—I can feel him strongly." She understood that she could meet her son's "rebirthable life" whenever she met recipients with a donor's organs. For her, the recipients' biologically "renewable life" and the donors' imaginary "rebirthable life" were equally valuable, and she felt she could communicate with both recipients' visible lives and donors' invisible lives.

6. "My Husband's Organ Donation Heals Me"

Mrs. Suzuki donated her husband's organ with a donation will of her husband, but felt that the two elements of her husband's death and her decision to donate his organs were separate. She also felt that reactions to organ donation for spouses and for children are different. "My husband died and left a donation will, so I donated his organ as a wife's mission. However, I could be against donation for my daughter's organs because children are a part of the mother's body. I feel emotional pain for my husband as a wife but I feel physical pain for my daughter as a mother." She does not feel "rebirthable life" for her husband but if she were to need to create "rebirthable life" for her daughter she might feel as other donor mothers do, that her daughter was reborn inside her.

1. Transplant surgeons understand the concept of donors' "rebirth-able life" metaphorically and see recipients' lives and donors' lives as separate (visible life vs. invisible life). According to their narratives, transplant surgeons have different individual perspectives, but their interpretations are in the abstract and not connected to their daily life, as are those of recipients and donor families.

2. Recipients' interpretations of donors' "rebirthable life" are based on their appreciation of their organ donations. Recipients have accepted donors' organs into their "renewable" bodies, so they feel donors' existences strongly inside themselves, and share the donors' "rebirthable life" in their imaginary world. Since they cannot help but feel guilt toward the donors' families, they attempt to obey what the donors would have wished for in life. A recipient's "renewable" body and a donor's "rebirthable life" live as life partners in one body, but are not equal: recipients are obedient to donors' "rebirthable life," which holds strong power to control them in their imaginary world.

3. Most donor families find it hard to accept the donor's death, since part of their body is still alive in their transplanted organ. As a result, they have created the "rebirthable life" of donors—from a partial organ to whole body in their imaginary world. This grows day by day for the donor family, and the donor's "rebirthable life" can have great power over the donor's bereaved family, and exists until the family members' deaths.

4. The new agent of the donor is very tricky to grasp because the character is ever-changing inside all concerned parties' imaginary world and controls them freely but strongly.

TRANSFORMING THE CONCEPT OF LIFE: MOVING FROM BIOLOGICALLY LIMITED LIFE TO IMAGINARY UNLIMITED LIFE

This chapter identified three terms created as a result of organ transplantation and developed by concerned parties—"gift of life," "renewable life," and "rebirthable life."

1. "Gift of life": all concerned parties had strong feelings about this phrase. Some transplant surgeons disliked it and felt it was rude toward donors and donor families, believing that "gift of love" would be more suitable. Some recipients were hesitant about the phrase, thinking that organ donation is much more precious behavior than just giving something. Most donor families also did not like the phrase because an organ is not a material item, and to them it is a way to keep the donor's life alive.

2. "Renewable life": this phrase also reflects different positions of concerned parties about an organ recipient's body and his/her bio-

logical or other life. However, the views focusing on both the limited biological visible human body and the unlimited imaginary invisible human existence are important interpretations in human society. Transplant surgeons use the phrase in their professional lives and their position is neutral. Recipients don't use this phrase solely for themselves but include donors because organ donation renews both donors and recipients. Donor families' reactions are opposite, as they think that recipients can renew their lives thanks to organ donation.

3. "Rebirthable life": this expresses the transformation in understanding of the concept of life for each category of concerned party. Transplant surgeons use "rebirthable life" for recipients rather than donors, as recipients are still alive as a result of the donors' deaths. Recipients use "rebirthable life" for both donors' and recipients' lives. Donor families feel that "rebirthable life" applies to donors, whose first life was biologically limited, but whose life has transferred to an imaginary unlimited life through organ donation.

The three phrases have been produced and developed as a result of organ transplantation issues, especially those concerning brain-dead donors. According to the interviewees' narrative data, all the concerned parties had new concepts of life and death, including the "gift of life," "renewable life," and "rebirthable life," whether consciously or not. However, their meanings and ways of using these terms are different, as reflected in their positions in relation to organ transplantation. Transplant surgeons' concept of life has transformed from one patient's life to two patients' lives together, which include a "renewable life" and a "rebirthable life." They give medical treatment to create a "renewable life" and they give thanks for the "rebirthable life." Recipients' concept of life has transformed to encompass both a biologically limited "renewable life" for recipients and an imaginary eternal "rebirthable life" for donors, living in parallel. Emerging medical technology has provided new information for donor families' concept of life: donors die once biologically and are reborn from a partial organ to a whole body in donor families' imaginary world, invisibly and eternally. Although donors no longer have an officially recognized life, all concerned parties nurture new and strong relationships with donors in an imaginary world, creating eternal life rather than just memories of the dead person. This "rebirthable life" needs a "renewable life" so that it can be reborn inside a recipient's body.

REFERENCES

Fox, R., and Swazey, J. (1992). *Spare Parts: Organ Replacement in American Society*. New York: Oxford University Press.

Lock, M. (2002). *Twice Dead: Organ Transplants and the Reinvention of Death*. Berkeley: University of California Press.

Mauss, M. (1954). *The Gift: Forms and Functions of Exchange in Archaic Societies*, translated by I. Cunnison. London: Cohen and West Ltd.

Namihira, E. (1996). *Cultural Anthropology of Life*. Tokyo: Shinchosha Co. Ltd.

Starzl, T. (1992). *The Puzzle People: Memories of a Transplant Surgeon*. Pittsburgh: University of Pittsburgh Press.

Yasuoka, M. K. (2006), "Rebirthable Life: Medical Anthropology Study of the Concept of Life According to Concerned Parties Involved in Brain Death and Organ Transplantation." PhD thesis: Department of History and Anthropology (Medical Anthropology), Graduate School of Letters, Hokkaido University, Sapporo, Japan (unpublished).

———. (2013). "Rebirthable Life: Narratives and Reproductive Life of Japanese Brain-Dead Donors." *Research Journal of Graduate Students of Letters* (Japan) 8, 73–81.

SEVEN

Conclusion

REBIRTHABLE LIFE

The previous chapters have introduced the different concepts of life among concerned parties to organ transplantation from brain-dead donors. Their narratives disclose their varied feelings about spending their daily lives involved with a donor's "rebirthable life." This conclusion considers the various broader issues associated with organ transplantation, which affect not only those parties directly involved but also many other people in this modern age who are users of emerging medical technology and must face the issues such innovations bring. I hope that my research is helpful in investigating the relationship between humans and such technology, taking into consideration the potential it offers both, benefit and harm, as well as the issues surrounding our moral and ethical responses to medical innovations and their results. It is imperative to discuss these topics, whether we are directly involved in organ transplantation or not: while transplant surgeons have made the decision to become concerned parties, the rest of us do not know whether or when we may become donors, recipients, or donor families. In this way we need to come to terms with current medical technology and prepare the way for our responses to emerging innovations.

My interview research revealed the simultaneous contradictory views held by concerned parties. Transplant surgeons consider themselves healers who save the lives of recipients, while at the same time they harvest organs from brain-dead patients, meaning that they cause these patients to lose their lives. Recipients are patients who accept organ transplantation gladly because of their medical conditions, while at the same time they gain an interdependent "transplanted life" and assume a reciprocal obligation to the sender of the "gift of life." And donor families

147

who donate their family member's organs feel that the donor has gained "rebirthable life," allowing them to try to continue their family relationships as before, while at the same time the bereaved family cremates the deceased's remains during the funeral process. In this way, transplant surgeons switch from painful feelings about a donor's death to joyful emotions at saving a recipient's life. Recipients, who have received transplanted organs to enable them to survive, sublimate their donors as targets of their gratitude in order to wipe out the guilt they feel at the deaths of the donors—as a result, they often try to extend and complete their lives to become donors themselves. Despite donor families' sense that donors' organs achieve "rebirthable life," which maintains the vital activities of the missing sons or daughters, they perform their duty of registering the donors' deaths as bereaved families.

Thus, donors have an ambivalent existence for all concerned parties, being at once living and dead and bringing both joy and sorrow, although the quality of happiness and sadness are surely different for each category of concerned party. The Japanese organ transplantation law both legalized and obscured the meaning of human death, stating, "Brain death is human death only if a person donates his/her organs." This created great confusion for transplant medical practice and concerned parties in Japan, but eventually transplant surgeons declared that brain death is human death. This meant that patients (recipients) could receive donated organs as a cure, and that bereaved families who offered organ donation now existed formally in the public eye as donor families, consistent with national policy.

In parallel, transplant surgeons receive hearts (physically and metaphorically) from brain-dead patients they cannot save, and mediate between these donors and recipients who can only survive with donated hearts; they support the recipients' lives with the donors' organs. Recipients feel that their donors have given them "love"—they make agreements with donors, whom they feel within their bodies, to fulfill their obligation in return by becoming donors themselves at the end of their second ("transplanted") life. Donor families feel that their children regain daily life with them, having received "rebirthable life" through their parents' decisions to donate and keep at least their organs alive. The concerned parties thus ensure the donors' existence in an imaginary invisible world. While in the real world, whether doctors, patients, or bereaved families, they live a life in which donors are only dead people to all nonconcerned parties, in their imaginary world donors are set in the center as still living people, and transplant surgeons, recipients, and donor families gather the threads of their various relationships with the donors' "rebirthable life." The concerned parties all seem to share an overlapping structure of this concept of life.

The interview research reveals certain phenomena that cannot be fully comprehended from the point of view that brain-dead organ transplantation is solely a medical treatment. This medical technology also acts as a device to bring to light a variety of other ethical and philosophical issues. The concerned parties' narratives include issues surrounding not only life and death but also concepts of "self" and "other." They show that organ transplantation has created a fluid relationship between living and dead people. Transplant surgeons tend to try to consider the various aspects of their roles as different entities, separating their care for the recipient through transplantation, their work with the donor family over agreement to donate and their harvesting of organs from brain-dead donors, and allocating the greatest burden of care to their (living) recipients. Recipients feel enormous appreciation for donors, but this can weaken over time if they go through retransplantation or re-retransplantation, and may lessen further with the progression of medical innovations that may not require human organs for donation. For donor families, however, the "rebirthable life" of their children as donors seems to last throughout their lifetime and does not change or receive less attention. Such differences in concerned parties' understanding of the role of donors create an issue about how we should understand the ambivalence of attitudes to donors. In other words, the relationship with donors continues to change considerably from day to day, depending on whether we understand that brain-dead donors are living or dead.

Transplant surgeons assess brain-dead transplantation as either something that should firmly be advocated or problematic medical care. Some practice happily in the belief that it is the best treatment they can offer their patients; others see it as a "best worst" option—the only current way to save their patients' lives—and hope that treatments such as xenotransplantation, regenerative medicine, or artificial organs will soon be developed, which may lessen the possibilities of organ rejection, as well as the need for organ harvesting. Transplant medical staff is not dissatisfied with the present organ transplantation technology, but nevertheless also keenly promote the development of new alternative technologies. When they refer to a "donor," they mean both donors they have been involved with as medics and future potential donors—that is, all donors who have contributed and will contribute to progress in medicine. When transplant surgeons speak of donors in general they talk about their medical contributions in a professional manner, but when referring to specific donors from whom they may have harvested organs, they talk about individual brain-dead and dying donors with much greater emotion.

Recipients have very little right to self-determination: they cannot choose whether their replacement organ comes from a donor who is dead or alive, and they have to maintain their dependent relationship with doctors in order to take immunosuppressive drugs to prevent organ rejection after transplant surgery. Once recipients start their "transplanted life," they have to continue the process of organ transplantation forever, whether via drugs or retransplantation: it pushes their bodies and becomes a habit, regardless of their will. In addition, if recipients repeat transplantation, the number of their "life-savers" continues to increase, and when the earlier transplanted organ is harvested to be replaced, that former donor's organ is no longer alive. Recipients do not forget their first donor after retransplantation, although the current donor becomes much more important as the "life" giver than the former one.

Donor families have only one donor: they do not experience large numbers of donors like transplant surgeons, or even perhaps two to three like some retransplant recipients. The "rebirthable life" of the donor via their organ inside a recipient's body is "eternal life" for their family. The donor family wants to insist that recipients take care of their loved one's organ and recipients feel that they are being watched by the donor family or living donor. Simultaneously, however, the donor's life is a "limited life," as the recipient's health affects the donated organ's life or death. Donor families live in a world where time stopped when they donated their family member's organ, and where the "rebirthable life" remains alive forever.

Concerned parties share donors' "rebirthable life" via organ donation, organ harvesting, and organ transplantation, but the relationships change as time passes. The nature of the relationships among transplant surgeons, recipients, donor families, and donors varies and has been developing within the large gaps at the boundary of donors' life and death. The differences are related to the various perspectives of the concerned parties, whether they focus on the "rebirthable life" of the donors or the "renewable life" taken over by the recipients.

Medical care surrounding brain-dead organ transplantation, one of the leading emerging medical technologies, has produced a wide variety of issues. First, a discussion of brain death involves the ambiguity surrounding the boundary between life and death: is a brain-dead person alive or dead, since their brain is dead but other parts of their body remain alive? In addition, the medical treatment that harvests a beating heart from a brain-dead person and transplants it into a patient enables this "other's" organ to cross the body's metaphorical border to be transplanted into the "self" of the recipient. As a result, concerned parties to organ transplantation—whether they like it or not—face issues of life and death. Brain-dead organ transplantation cannot take place unless donors' brain death is regarded as human death, although this is currently unclear in Japanese law; recipients are facing death—when offered a transplant their choice is to take it or to die; likewise, transplant surgeons have the skill to save their patients through transplantation when no alternative successful medical treatments are available. The Japan Organ Transplant Network (JOTN) is desperate to distribute donor cards, but they produce no substantive result because the "life" during which a person fills in his/her donation will and the "life" during which his/her family consents to organ donation are supported by entirely different concepts of life. A living person considers his/her own death as just a metaphysical future event occurrence, while a bereaved family sees the death of a relative as a present event with immense sadness and pain. Brain death becomes the obvious boundary between a living and a dead person: a relatively new criterion generated by advances in modern medicine. Brain-dead donors become involved in the living arena again via their organs transplanted into the recipients' bodies, creating difficult challenges for all concerned, on which continuing discussion is absolutely necessary.

The concerned parties also cannot avoid considering issues surrounding "self" and "other" through organ transplantation. Recipients experience at first hand the "invasion" of their bodies by others' organs. Conversely, the donor's organs are now able to cross the border into another's body via medical technology. From whichever perspective is considered, all concerned parties are affected by this blurring of the lines between "self" and "other." As described earlier, these cross-border organs are admired as "reviving medical treatment" to save dying recipients' lives and are considered the "gift of life" of donors, filled with altruism. For bereaved families who have suffered the brain death of a relative, organ transplantation fulfills their dearest wish, which is to keep their loved one alive; donor families are also heralded as "silent heroes." Organ transplantation has led to a hybridization of the human body, creating an ambiguous boundary between self and other, and making it possible to cross this frontier. And donors' organs have become medical resources for recipients, creating the challenge of an interdependent relationship between recipients and donors (and donor families), through which recipients' bodies become containers of "rebirthable life" (see figure 7.1).

As seen above, emerging medical technologies have given "rebirthable biological life" to patients awaiting death, and continue to reshape and redefine the impossible. On the other hand, they have created brain-dead patients whose brains are no longer functioning but whose hearts are still beating. Although donors gain an imaginary "rebirthable life" and a new existence through organ donation, it is impossible for them to recover a "rebirthable biological life" with current medicine. Medical care to protect people's lives that relies on a treatment strategy targeting human organs as medical resources is therefore a cutting-edge technology that defies the boundaries and limitations of contemporary medicine. Further developments in medicine, such as regenerative medicine, are also expected to lead to recovery of brain function or avoidance of loss of brain function. However, the further research into these new technologies progresses, the clearer it becomes it will be many years before they will be ready for clinical application, despite the potential options being numerous. As this book has illustrated, by focusing on a medical treat-

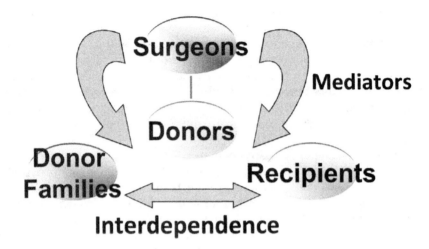

Figure 7.1.   Rebirthable Life

ment that continues to improve and a concept of life that keeps transforming, it is important for us to pay attention to the relationship between cutting-edge medical care and society's needs in the future.

Afterword

My father passed away suddenly of a heart attack at 20:00 on August 13, 2014 at home in Japan while I was writing the final manuscript of this book. He was in the bathtub when it happened and I was the first person to find his body: my mother and I pulled him out of the bathtub and I gave him cardiac massage while we waited for the police and ambulance. Once I thought I heard his voice, but it was just air and his chest never rose again with breath. He passed away forty minutes before I found him; it appears that he had suffered a heart attack and drowned. When the police and emergency paramedics arrived, they took my father to the hospital of my home university, so I took my mother (who is blind in one eye and relied heavily on my father's support) in the hope that my father would survive miraculously but it was not to be.

I wondered whether, if my father had been young and had made an organ donation will, my mother and I could have made a level-headed decision about organ donation automatically in the ambulance, even while I tried to comfort her. My father had had a stroke due to an irregular heartbeat from thyroid failure twenty-eight years earlier, before I entered university for my undergraduate studies. At that time I was in a panic and in tears every day, but he survived with a pacemaker for twenty-eight years and lived to be eighty-seven, which is more than ten years longer than the average Japanese man's life-span. My mother and I often talk about my father's death. Without him we are lonely but not sad: he had a long life and my mother did her best for him and for my older sister and me too. We wondered about organ donation, though. As a researcher, leading interviews with informants and trying to understand their experience of their world, I learned a lot and thought that I understood their narratives. But after losing my father I recognized that I had not fully understood their descriptions. Donor families insist on the importance of a donor's donation will; while I understood the surface of their narratives, now I understand what they really wanted to tell me: the bereaved family has no way of truly knowing the deceased's wishes and can only guess and surmise from their own knowledge. On losing a family member our feelings are in immense flux and we cannot confirm whether our guesses are correct unless we have written proof from the dead person in the form of a donation will. Organ donation issues require both a subjective view and an objective view to make an informed decision.

JAPANESE FUNERAL CULTURE

I had always assumed that the low numbers of organ donations in Japan were connected to the Japanese concepts of death and the dead body. Through the experience of my father's death, I started to research Japanese funeral culture such as traditions, rituals, customs, beliefs, and similar, to imagine the emotional aspects experienced by donor families, hoping that this would help me to understand the irreplaceable elements of donor families' grieving processes and their world. Although I am a Japanese anthropologist, this was my first time participating in a Buddhist funeral. My father came to Japan from Russia when he was twenty-three years old and became a Japanese Samurai: he was an instructor of *kendo* [art of Japanese fencing], *iaido* [art of drawing the Japanese sword], *kyudo* [art of Japanese archery], and others. His younger sister emigrated to the United States, so he had no family in Japan and no other attendees from his side of the family at his funeral. In addition, my mother and I are Christian (Christians make up 1 percent of the total population of Japan), so I have very little knowledge of Buddhism and Shinto (the predominant religion in Japan is a syncretization of Shinto with Buddhism).

Understanding the reticence felt by Japanese donor families toward organ donation and the long, complex, and metaphysical grieving processes requires knowledge of and a cultural perspective on Japanese funerals. In my research I understood those Japanese recipients' deep appreciation of and strong feelings of guilt toward the donor and donor family (especially compared with recipients in other countries), as well as the low rate of organ donations were connected to Japanese funeral culture and the concept of the dead body. In fact, while many specialists say that the low rate of organ donations in Japan is due to cultural barriers, nobody has outlined what these cultures or barriers are, and nobody has set out specific reasonable answers for the lack of donations. I agree that organ transplantation is related to cultural issues, but although I have been searching for years for a specific reason I haven't found it yet. I think that studying the attitudes of bereaved families may help researchers to understand organ donation issues from the perspectives of donor families, recipients, and transplant surgeons.

Elements of a Japanese Funeral

The Japanese funeral has three elements: *noukan* [encoffinment], *tsuya* [wake] and *sougi* [funeral service].[1] These usually take place over three days.

1. *Noukan* is a ritual washing of the coffined dead body and preparing it in the burial outfit for travel to Jodo (the "pure land," paradise, or Buddhist heaven).
2. *Tsuya* is the last night to say goodbye to the deceased: family members and relatives gather around the dead body to talk and share reminiscences all night (a memorial vigil or wake).
3. *Sougi* is part of the funeral ritual that consoles the spirits of the dead person, not only for family and relatives but also for colleagues and the local community.

DIVERSITY OF JAPANESE FUNERAL TRADITIONS ACCORDING TO REGION, AGE, AND SOCIAL CONDITION

Japanese funeral culture has experienced change in recent years, becoming less traditional and exhibiting more personal values. Some elements—such as the participants' region, age, and social condition—are strongly connected with such phenomena. As a result, it has become difficult to give an example of a "typical" Japanese funeral.

1. Region

Japan is a small narrow country made up of several islands: its total land area is similar to that of California State, but the Japanese coastline is longer than the American coastline and the country contains different climates, lifestyles, and cultures. Southwest and northeast Japan have different funeral customs—strongly traditional in the southwest but

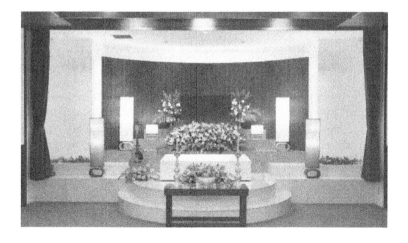

Ceremonial Hall Where My Father's *Tsuya* [wake] and *Sougi* [funeral service] Were Held Aoyagi Ceremonial Hall website.

more mixed with those of other cultures and nationalities in the northeast. My home is in northern Japan, where ceremonies tend to be very rational and simple because many people emigrated from the main island to Hokkaido (the northern island), which contains a mix of different cultures. For example, in the mainland area of Japan (including Tokyo in the east and Osaka in the west), only family and relatives are invited to *tsuya*, while everyone is invited to *sougi*, thus dividing the family and public elements of the ritual. On Hokkaido (which includes Sapporo), on the other hand, everyone who is available is invited to both *tsuya* and *sougi*: since the population is made up of immigrants from all parts of Japan, the mix of regional cultures tends to lead people to band together to help each other out.

2. Age

Japanese funeral style has recently undergone changes (and this trend seems likely to continue as the twenty-first century progresses), transforming from a more traditional style to one allowing greater expression of individuality. Another aspect of this transformation is strongly reflected in the swift advance of globalization in Japan as people gain knowledge from different countries and their cultures through the internet and other technologies. At the same time, Japanese traditional local culture and beliefs still remain deeply rooted in the countryside within Japan. Japanese people love learning about new cultures and trends from Western countries, yet they also feel the pull of the traditional and old-fashioned cultural background in Eastern countries.

3. Social Condition

During World War II, many young sons were drafted and died in the war for Japan, and their mothers received only a piece of paper (a war death notice) announcing the loss. The young man's family, other soldiers and public officials gave three rousing cheers for the sacrifice for the Japanese nation, offering a smile and congratulations. Nevertheless, every mother must feel sorrow at losing a beloved son; while smiling on the outside they were secretly crying at home alone at night. At that time, a funeral was performed without the remains of the war dead, so the mother would hold an urn in which was placed the death notice instead the ashes of her son. Such were the losses sustained in World War II that, although showing sadness and crying in public were still frowned on by traditional thinkers, the barriers began to break down and shows of grief outside the home became more accepted.

THE MODERN JAPANESE FUNERAL SERVICE:
MOVING FROM COMMUNITY VALUES TO INDIVIDUALITY

The trend toward a more individualistic and domestic funeral has become increasingly common in Japan. As a result, the role of funeral culture has also changed, moving from a public social display enabling society to recognize and support bereaved people (Japan had no welfare service before World War II, so it was important for the wider family and community to support bereaved people who might have lost their family's breadwinner) to giving greater importance to personal preferences. The family funeral is becoming more popular than the public, in keeping with the preferences of the deceased and their family; some people are now preparing their own funerals while still young and healthy to enable their desires to be registered. Not only the whole funeral service but also individual aspects of funerals have been emphasized in the creation of individual preferences, such as the use of a portrait of the deceased person at a gathering rather than a formal funeral service.

CASE STUDY: MY FATHER'S FUNERAL (AUGUST 13–16, 2014,
SAPPORO, JAPAN)

My father[2] passed away on August 13, 2014, in Sapporo (in northern Japan—the least traditional island) and we held his funeral ceremony for four days (in fact, in total it took fifty-two days until my father could be

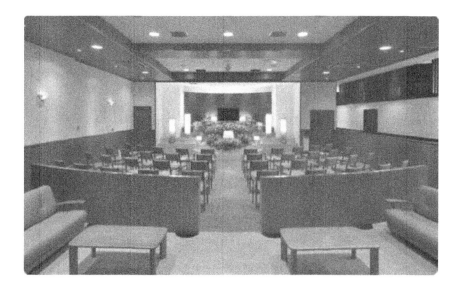

Family Funeral Room Aoyagi Ceremonial Hall website.

laid in his grave alongside his parents, brothers, and sisters). We had a family funeral because he had retired and all his brothers, sisters, and friends living in Japan had already passed away, so only my mother's relatives attended his funeral. The bereaved close family members included his wife (my mother), his elder daughter (my sister) with her husband and their two sons, and his youngest daughter (myself).

We decided on the funeral hall in the hospital where my father was taken. Our choice was very simple: Aoyagi Ceremonial Hall is the closest such venue to my home. When I called the hall, they came to the hospital promptly with two cars: one a hearse carrying my father's casket and the other an ordinary car for my mother and me. My father's body was placed in the casket; my mother and I were driven to my home and my sister's family followed in their car. When we got home two *noukan-shi* [layers-out] placed my father's body in a prepared coffin with dry ice and ritual products and they performed a simple ritual for a dead person. Now my father's life was over and we had started the Buddhist ritual for him to go to heaven.

August 13–15: My Father's Noukan [encoffinment]

Because my father passed away from a heart attack in the bathtub it was considered a drowning incident: I was interviewed by the police as a witness at the scene because I was the person who discovered the body. I explained that when I got home from university at 19:45, my father was taking a bath. I tried to wait for him to finish as I planned to take a bath as soon as possible afterwards because it was mid-summer. I waited fifty-five minutes, but thought that he was taking longer than usual, so I knocked on the door at 20:40. Receiving no response I went in and saw that he had sunk and was lying on the bottom of bathtub. I shouted out, "Mom, Dad is drowning! Come on!" and I called the police and ambulance. I performed heart massage but he never breathed again.

We took him to my university's hospital and an ER doctor asked us, "Shall we stop heart massage? Look at the vital signs on the monitor." The monitor showed that he had flat-lined and he was moved to the mortuary with a white cloth covering his face. I took this off and rubbed my cheek against his: it was as cold as ice. His body was then moved into a casket. The next day, August 14, was *tomobiki* [pulling friends]—a day in the six-day Buddhist cycle on which one's luck affects that of one's friends, which is therefore auspicious for weddings but to be avoided for funerals—which extended the funeral period from three to four days. Our priest visited my home and performed *Makura-gyo* ["pillow service": chanting by a Buddhist priest]. I spent time with my father's body all day, replacing the candlelight whenever it went out and offering incense. His face was so peaceful and this helped to heal my grief.

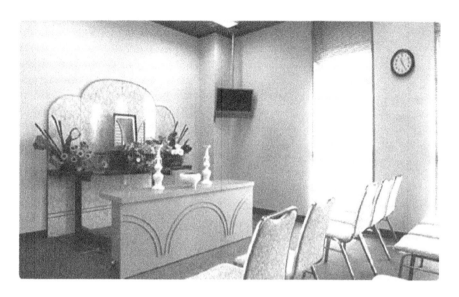

Makura-gyo ["Pillow Service": Chanting by a Buddhist Priest] Aoyagi Ceremonial Hall website. Note: My father was laid out in his own bed at home and our priest performed this ceremony with my mother and me early in the morning the day after his death because we had space in our house. However, most Japanese people live in relatively small apartments and may not have space, so the ceremonial hall rents this room for **makura-gyo**.

August 15: My Father's Tsuya *[wake]*

In the morning, a *noukan-shi* [layer-out] came to my home and performed a ritual called *yukan* [washing a dead body for burial]. He washed my father's body, then he called my mother, sister, and me, and handed us a wet paper towel each to wipe the body. My mother wiped his legs and whispered, "You used to be a person of sinews but your knees became so skinny, honey." My elder sister wiped his hands and whispered, "You worked very hard for us with these hands, Dad." I wiped his face and complained "Dad, everybody says that my face is copy of yours, but I wanted to be a beautiful woman!" The *noukan-shi* dressed my father in a white kimono and *tabi* [Japanese socks] and held a stick to my father's hand with some coins for crossing death's river and his favorite items to keep him from feeling lonely. In the afternoon, we said goodbye to my father and he left the home he had built in 1978 and moved to the funeral hall.

His *tsuya* started at 16:00. My family and my mother's relatives came together for the priest's reading of the sutras and incense-burning by all the audience. Our priest said some words about my father and I greeted the audience in my mother's place; then we had dinner, reminiscing together about our memories of my father. Some neighbors also came and signed the condolence book at the front desk in the funeral hall. Nine relatives spent the night in individual rooms in the funeral hall; my mother and her elder sister spent the night in a twin bedroom. My elder sister, brother-in-law, and I slept together in one room and took turns watching my father overnight. I was typing this book beside him because he hated to disturb my research and I felt that he was happy for me to keep working. His face was the most handsome I have ever seen it that night.

August 16: My Father's Sougi *[funeral service]*

On the morning of August 16, my sister, her husband, and I made coffee and served it to everyone who spent time at the funeral hall and kept chatting about my father's memory. We all had breakfast together. At 10:00, my father's *sougi* started with our priest's reading of the sutras and incense-burning by all the audience.[3] The priest told another story about my father, and then his funeral service was over. At 11:00, my father's hearse left the funeral hall, so the audience took a bus together to the crematorium. My mother was holding an *ihai* [spirit tablet] (a wooden board on which is written the posthumous Buddhist name of the deceased, which will be kept at home after the funeral) with my support (she needs a stick to walk) and my sister was holding a photograph of our father.

We arrived at the crematorium as *kugiuti* [coffin nailing] started and we had to say our final goodbye. My father looked as if he was only sleeping and likely to wake up from his nap, but this miracle never happened. My mother put his favorite book into his coffin; I put in a walnut he used for finger rehabilitation after his stroke. My brother-in-law put in a bamboo sword because my father was a grand master of *kendo* [art of Japanese fencing], my older nephew put in a caramel, which his grandfather had always given him as a little boy, and my younger nephew put in an *orizuru* [origami crane], which his grandfather had taught him to make. Then his coffin was closed and nailed and he was cremated. His wife (my mother) squeezed my hand.

The family and relatives then moved to a waiting room and had a rest while my sister and I went shopping to buy many bottles of tea and juice for lunch. On the way to the shop we passed a huge Japanese garden and met my uncle, who took a picture of us as a memorial for the day of the funeral. We went back to the waiting room and had a traditional Buddhist vegetarian and chatted about dead people in our family—not only my father but others too. My brother-in-law and I went to the city hall and had to request the death certificate and certificate of cremation within seven days of his death: there was a lot of tough paperwork to complete during that short period. Then my father became cremains.

Kotsuage then started and we formed a line to welcome my father's skeleton as it appeared. The crematorium worker crushed his skull and other bones—he had strong bones and teeth so many remained clearly visible. She picked up his special bone—*nodo-botoke* [Adam's apple]—and put it into a small reliquary, which my mother kept carefully. Then we picked up as many as possible of my father's bones with chopsticks and put them into a big reliquary, which my sister kept. My mother whispered, "Now, honey, you have become dead burned bones!" We drove back to the funeral hall, where the priest read the sutras, told another story about my father and left. I gave the concluding funeral speech in my mother's place and my father's funeral was over.

I recorded all the events of my father's funeral in field notes as an anthropologist because the priest told me, "Your father had been worried about you, Maria, but he was so happy to tell me you got your PhD. Although you had no job for a long time, when you got your grant in 2014 your father told me about it and said, 'My youngest daughter finally got a big grant and became an anthropologist. I'm a grand master of *kendo* [art of Japanese fencing] and came from Russia to Japan when I was twenty-three years old, but my youngest daughter who is a little rambunctious youngster finally outdid her parents!' Your face is the image of your father's so you should be a grand master of anthropology instead of *kendo*!"

SEPTEMBER 30: *SHIJYU-KU NICHI HOUYO* [RITUAL MEAL OF THE FORTY-NINTH DAY]

On this day finally the deceased goes to Buddhist heaven: a photograph decorated with flowers and the funeral urn with an *ihai* [spirit tablet] are put on the altar beside the family altar. Then the bereaved family celebrates the deceased leaving for heaven with a *hoyo-zen* [Buddhist memorial service meal] with close family members.

It takes forty-nine days (seven times seven) for a deceased person to go to Buddhist heaven. August 19 was the ceremony of the seventh day after my father's death, at which our priest read the sutras and told a story about my father, and my mother, my sister's family, and I had a sushi party for lunch. We skipped the ceremonies on August 26, September 2, September 9, September 16, and September 23 (the succeeding seven-day intervals after his death), then the ceremony of the forty-ninth day after my father's death arrived on September 30. Our priest read the sutras and told another story about my father. My mother, my sister's family (except my younger nephew who lives in Kyoto as his university term had started) and some relatives came to my home and after the ceremony we had a sushi party. Finally, my father could go to Buddhist heaven.

On October 3, the Ministry of Foreign Affairs of Japan granted us temporary permission to inter my father's bones in the family grave. Because he came to Japan from Russia at twenty-three, he was present in the *koseki* [official family registry] but there was no record of his birth and life up to the age of twenty-three in Japan; thus, my mother could not claim my father's grave and his ashes and bones could not be placed in a tomb.[4] We still have some tough paperwork with Ministry of Foreign Affairs of Japan to make the permission permanent.

Finally my father could be interred on October 3 and his *kaimyo* [posthumous Buddhist name] was listed on his tombstone. Our priest, my mother, my sister's family, and I gathered at his tombstone as the priest read the sutras. And at last my father's funeral ritual was over.

JAPANESE FUNERAL BELIEFS AND ORGAN TRANSPLANTATION ISSUES

My father passed away suddenly as I was writing this book and I had to take a long bereavement leave. While I originally had no plan to write about my father's death in my book on organ transplantation issues, after the event I found myself considering organ donation many times, partly through discussions with family members who were aware of my field of research (although in fact my father was too old to donate and could not because he had a heart attack). My research has involved concerned parties to organ donation (especially donor families), and when I lost my own father I felt that I could understand the feelings of bereaved families in a similar situation, even though no organ donation was possible in my case. I therefore decided to introduce Japanese funeral culture to the audience of this book, to show that our very traditional funeral beliefs still remain intact in modern Japanese society.

NOUKAN-SHI: SPECIALISTS IN THE PSYCHOLOGICAL STATUS OF BEREAVED FAMILIES

This was my first opportunity to meet and talk with *noukan-shi* [layers-out] directly. Public awareness of *noukan-shi* rose following the 2008 Japanese movie *Okuribito* [Departures], after which every Japanese person knew the name of *okuribito*, which describes the work of *noukan-shi*, although most did not know much about the role itself, and nor did I. When I met and spent some days with them I noticed that they are specialists in dealing with bereaved families, especially their psychological status. They understand very well how much a bereaved family needs grief care and they know though their experience what to do to assuage their sadness and help them to recover from the shock of their family member's death.

THE *NOUKAN-SHI'S* RITUAL PERFORMANCE *YUKAN* [WASHING A DEAD BODY FOR BURIAL]

1. Praying and greeting the deceased with respect to begin *yukan*
2. Embalming the face with *fukumi-wata* (wiping the dead person's mouth with cotton) and shaving or applying make-up to make the face peaceful
3. Washing the body and changing the clothes to veil the skin
4. Supporting the dead person's preparation for the journey to heaven

I found watching the *yukan* ritual at home for my father's dead body very impressive: this ritual respects not only the dead person but also the bereaved family members. A *noukan-shi* has to create an atmosphere of both solemnity for the deceased and sympathy for the bereaved family, healing them by respecting their loss. Water has great importance for Japanese society, owing to the geographical nature of the country, which is formed of several islands surrounded by ocean. Water is a holy item for Japanese people, and it is used in *yukan* by the *noukan-shi* and family members to purify the deceased not only physically but also in preparing the soul for heaven. This participatory funeral ritual helps the bereaved family cleanse the body physically and also experience their last communication with the deceased, allowing them to bid their loved one farewell.

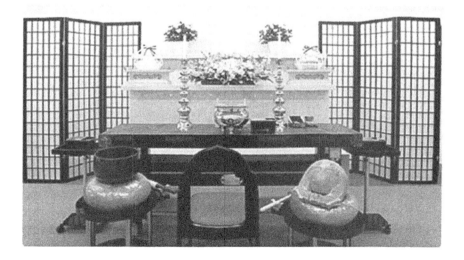

Saidan [Funeral Altar after *Yukan*] Aoyagi Ceremonial Hall website

NARRATIVE OF *NOUKAN-SHI* LEADER (PRESIDENT OF THE FUNERAL HALL) CONCERNING ORGAN TRANSPLANTATION

I asked to interview the *noukan-shi* to learn about his specialist knowledge of bereavement and to investigate his opinions about organ donation and organ transplantation issues. He told me how important a dead person's will is for the bereaved family (such as a living will, organ donation will, etc.). Because the dead cannot speak, bereaved family members can only guess at the deceased's will and preferences, but they really want to honor these as much as possible even though consensus may only be reached after a long and tough time.

I offered to interview one of the *noukan-shi* who administered my father's funeral rituals. He recommended that I speak to the president of the funeral hall because he not only respected him as the president of his company but was also proud of him as a person. He arranged the interview and I learned many things about matters of life and death and the president's opinions about organ transplantation issues. I thought that he would have negative feelings toward organ harvesting, but his answer was, "I think that it is wonderful thing!" I asked him why he felt this. He told me: "If the dead person has a donation will and the bereaved family members understand this and inform the medical staff, they feel that they can make their lost family member's organ donation will come true; in addition, some seriously ill patient's life could be saved. That's a really wonderful thing. I agree with the idea of organ donation!"

EXPANDING MY ANTHROPOLOGICAL RESEARCH: LEARNING FROM MY LATE FATHER

Through my experience of my father's sudden death I learned many things and gained insight into the plight of bereaved families who have to make swift choices on behalf of their dead loved ones. I list some of the main details below to further my own research and in a wish to contribute to future medical anthropological research about organ transplantation.

A. Unconscious Patients' Family and Organ Donation

Most brain-dead donors are unconscious patients in the ER and cannot provide information about their donation preferences unless they keep a donor card about them, on which the details of their donation will are clearly set out. At that time, the patient's family is in a panic and under extreme emotional stress, so transplant surgeons or ER doctors should not offer organ donation at this stage, even though they need fresh organs, unless the patient has a donor card; the offer might make family members fear that their loved one is likely to receive less life-sustaining care. After organ donation, the donor family's grief becomes more complex and deeper and if they feel they have been coerced into donating their loved one's organs, it can cause serious psychological problems later. Discussion of organ donation should not put pressure on the families of seriously ill patients.

B. Psychological Aspects of Bereaved Families

All donor families except those of living donors are bereaved families and organ donations rely on their agreement to organ harvesting from the dead patient. Most research about organ donation issues focuses on the donor, but at the time of organ donation the donor has usually already lost consciousness or died, so medical staff have to respect the bereaved family's judgment concerning organ donation, taking into account their psychological responses.

C. Various Thoughts of Donor Families

Most donor families hope that the recipient will gain good health and a long life because the bereaved want to feel that their lost family member is helping someone after death. This comforts them, and some bereaved family members think that the deceased lives on inside the recipient. Nevertheless, different donor families make their decisions to donate their loved ones' organs based on different factors and have a variety of reactions to recipients after the transplant has taken place, so it cannot be assumed that they all feel happy about the donation or wish to hear from the recipient.

D. Organ Donation Will as a Living Will

According to my data, an organ donation will is a significant component of bereavement care for donor families. The president of a Japanese funeral hall, a *noukan-shi* and specialist in the care of bereaved families, agreed that an organ donation will is very important: even after struggling with their loved one's loss, the bereaved family members want to respect the deceased's will. We should learn from his words and advocate that everyone should indicate their intention of organ donation to each one of their family members and make their preferences well known.

Finally, I would like to add my own information through my experience of losing my father. With or without organ donation, losing a family member is very sad and difficult to accept, and we struggle to create meaning and place individual interpretations on a loved one's death. I wondered many times about what my reaction would have been if my father had been offered organ donation—if he were much younger and in better health when he died—but I couldn't find the answer, even though I have been researching the field (through the narratives of transplant surgeons, recipients, and donor families) since 2000. Before this event, I could not fully understand concerned parties' true feelings, but now I can tell that if my father had had a donor card and we, his family, knew his organ donation will, we would definitely have donated his organs because we love him and we would have wanted to make his wish come true.

During the writing this book I lost my father but I gained new field of research: the specialist arena of bereaved family care, such as Japanese *noukan-shi* and similar. Expanding the knowledge in this field will contribute to research into both organ donation issues and grief care for donor families.

NOTES

1. I learned all the special terms and explanations of Japanese funeral culture from interviews with the president of Ceremony Hall Aoyagi and staff.

2. My father came to Japan in 1950, arriving at Hokkaido, which is very close to Russia. In 1975 we moved to Sapporo, the fifth biggest city in Japan (population almost 2 million) in north-east Japan. Many people settled here from Honshu (the main island) and the southwestern islands in the nineteenth and twentieth centuries, so the weight of tradition is lower and the atmosphere is freer than in other parts of Japan. The closest beach to Sapporo is the location of the "Wada case" of 1968.

3. Funeral attendees bring money (*Koden* or ["flower fee"]) and the bereaved family sends a *Koden-gaeshi* [gift in return for a funeral offering] after the funeral. This is usually a small present such as sweets, coffee, or sometimes a gift voucher; roasted laver (*Yaki-nori*) and green tea (*Ryoku-tya*) are the most common. However this strong Japanese custom of traditional exchanges is highlighted by Margaret Lock, a prominent medical anthropologist, as one of the reasons the country has such a low rate of organ donations.

4. The bereaved family is invited by their priest to perform the ceremony at the graveyard (the funeral payment is known as the "flower fee"). My sister arranged flowers for my father's grave for him and his parents. They were beautiful and included lilies (white chrysanthemums are traditional flowers for funerals in Japan but recently white lilies and other softly colored flowers are in use, although roses and other flowers with thorns are avoided).

Appendix

The Japanese organ transplantation law is strongly linked to organ dona-tion numbers in the country. While on the surface Japan is a very modern country, internally many people cling to traditional values and long-standing cultural beliefs that have been passed down through genera-tions about life, death, the afterlife, and so on. These attitudes are also deeply connected to the motivations of Japanese donors and donor fami-lies when deciding whether to create an organ donation will or to donate their brain-dead family member's organs. The law itself is also greatly influenced by the tradition and culture associated with the Japanese con-cept of life and death, which is shared by other Far Eastern countries such as China and Korea. Nevertheless Japanese organ donation numbers are extremely low compared with other Far Eastern countries. Indeed, Japan has the lowest organ donation rate in the world.

The original Japanese organ transplantation law was established very late in comparison with other countries, even though Japan is a highly medically advanced country. This was the result of the "Wada case," as Dr. Lock, a medical anthropologist, pointed out (Lock 2002). The original law was implemented in 1997; it was partly revised in January 2010, and completely revised in July 2010. The following sections summarize the main points of the law, showing how the "Wada case" had both adverse impacts and positive effects.

THE ORIGINAL JAPANESE ORGAN TRANSPLANTATION LAW
(OCTOBER 16, 1997–JULY 16, 2010)

After a long intermission following the "Wada case" in 1968, the first Japanese organ transplantation law was implemented on October 16, 1997. Various parties who had advocated organ transplantation had wait-ed a long time for the law and expected brain-dead transplantation to begin as soon as possible, but it was not in fact put to use for a further two years: the second heart transplant in Japan was performed on Febru-ary 28, 1999 (thirty-one years after the first). This was the country's first brain-dead transplant, with brain-death tests conducted under the new law.

One reason for the low organ donation numbers in Japan is that the original Japanese organ transplantation law was one of the strictest in the world in three main ways.

1. Brain Death

The law stated that only when patients had consented to donate their organs would brain-dead status be recognized as the death of the body (brain death thus becoming legal death only in that circumstance). This gave rise to the ambiguity contained in the two definitions of death in Japan: those prepared to donate their organs died from brain death; those choosing not to died from heart death. This criterion seems to have given a negative impression to Japanese people and, as a result, social consensus on brain death has not yet been reached. In addition, all topics surrounding death are still a social and cultural deep-seated taboo in Japan. The resulting confusion has caused great anxiety over organ donation in the country.

2. Organ Donation Will

Japanese people were required by the law to have both an organ donation will and the consent of their family for the donation. This made it particularly difficult to ensure that organs would be donated if a patient became brain-dead. Even if the patient had a current donor card, if their family member was against organ donation then the organs could not be donated and the donation will was useless. This removed the right to self-determination. Similarly, if the family agreed to the donation but the brain-dead patient did not have a donor card (or gave any indication that they were against organ donation) the family could not donate the organs. Since it was unusual to have both the necessary donation will and the family's consent, this aspect of the law offered the field of organ transplantation little or no progress.

3. Age Limit

The original law prohibited organ donation from children under the age of fifteen years. As a result, organs were denied to recipient candidate children within Japan. All young recipients were thus entirely reliant on living donors within their family circle—for the most part their mother, father, or siblings—if any were a suitable match. All heart recipient candidate children had to go abroad if they were to receive a donated organ. The World Health Organization (WHO), however, called for organ self-sufficiency to reduce international trafficking in human tissues and organs, and organizing an overseas transplant became more difficult. In addition, every country in the world was facing its own severe organ shortage, so none had the capacity to supply other countries' recipient candidates. There was therefore little or no hope that recipient candidate children could survive.

THE REVISED LAW (JULY 17, 2010 TO PRESENT)

Once the first law was established, everybody expected (especially transplant surgeons and recipient candidates) that organ transplant operations would now be possible for recipients so that they could receive an organ from a brain-dead donor. Concerned parties pinned all their hopes the new law. Most other Japanese people (those with no connection to organ donation) also believed that advanced medical technology had reached a pinnacle and thought that the "gift of life" had provided freedom from organ failure for future patients. Nevertheless, organ donation numbers in Japan remained the lowest and the organ shortage the most severe in the world, and many Japanese people still relied on overseas transplants. Although the medical world was changing rapidly, Japanese people were still relying on overseas transplants and living donors within the family circle.

The first Japanese organ transplantation law had many serious problems and a plan was put in place to revise it three years later in 2000, but this was repeatedly postponed so that the revision did not take place until 2010. During these thirteen years, Japanese people seemed slowly to be accepting both brain death and organ transplantation. However, in retrospect it appears that they were in fact just becoming accustomed to the terminology rather than accepting the details and changing their concept of life and death more fully. In other words, Japanese people began to take the terms "brain death," "organ transplantation," and "organ donation" for granted, but still considered them somebody else's problems, about which they did not need to concern themselves too deeply. There is still a huge gap in understanding and approach between concerned parties to organ transplantation and others: organ transplantation issues are vital problems for concerned parties, but may sound like morbid topics to others and be considered ill-omened matters within traditional thought in Japan.

The revised organ transplantation law brought in three main changes to the original.

1. A Vaguer Standard of Brain Death

The revised law did not put much emphasis on the big issue of brain death, especially on whether the definition of brain death was indeed human death. (A discussion of brain death is still ongoing in the country, not only debating the definition but also examining various arguments concerning the perspective and attitudes of Japanese people and society.) The revision deleted the original statement that brain death was human death only in the case that the patient had agreed to donate their organs, but it stated neither that brain death was human death nor that it was not. The revised law was based on the assumption that public under-standing had been spreading among Japanese people, but that may or may not be true. Many people recognized the new law without any argu-ment, and it seemed that brain death might have become accepted as a definition of human death in Japan, but the evidence in ensuing years shows that this is not the case.

2. *Organ Donation Wills and Family-Presumed Consent*

The revised organ transplantation law permitted organ harvesting in two situations:

1. if the donor had declared via a paper-based organ donation will that they wished to donate their organs and the bereaved family did not refuse, or there was no close family; or
2. if the donor had no organ donation will but the bereaved family had a paper-based declaration of intent in which they consented to donate their family member's organs.

The biggest change was that, as long as the patient did not refuse to donate, the family's consent was presumed; this restored to some extent the right of the individual to self-determination. The meaning of family "consent" was very vague, however, predominantly because the defini-tion of family itself was not set out: who counts as a family member— does it include legal family or only blood family, and how closely relat-ed? While parents and children are blood family, for example, husbands and wives are not. In addition, the notion of "family" is becoming in-creasingly complex in the modern age, with the addition of step-children, step-siblings, and similar. It was hoped that family members knew of the donor's organ donation will and supported it, but if they held the oppo-site view to the patient, their decision would still outweigh the individu-al's organ donation will (or indeed the individual's refusal to donate an organ).

3. *Repeal of Age Limit*

Under the revised law organs could be donated from a child under the age of fifteen years if the family had a paper-based declaration of intent. (To be precise, this could only occur after the twelfth week of life once the organs were sufficiently developed.) This change offered children a chance to donate organs, but as they were still under the legal age of consent their family members (usually their parents) would be the decision makers. It also meant that a recipient candidate child, especially a heart recipient candidate, had the opportunity to receive organs in Japan rather than relying on an overseas organ transplant or a living donor inside family circle. This was a response to WHO's policy of attaining national organ self-sufficiency to reduce organ trafficking.

The revised organ transplantation law offered a more positive legal basis for recipients, but some people have strong doubts about whether it is in fact better than the original and are not entirely convinced by it. In the year of the law's revision (2010) the number of organ donations in Japan jumped up about eight- or nine-fold, and has since remained stable, but it is not clear that the revised law is as successful as had been hoped. The definition of death and the position of brain death remain very vague, and many conflicting interpretations are available. While the patient's own decision to donate organs is very important, family-presumed consent is now more effective in increasing numbers of organ donations. There is concern about whether the current law will in fact increase organ donations from donors with donation wills and reflect the right of self-determination based on altruism; that is, the "gift of life," which is the fundamental philosophy of organ donation.

Now that the age limit has been repealed, children under the age of fifteen years have the opportunity to donate or receive organs. The original age limit meant that other countries, such as the United States, Australia, and Germany, kindly accepted young Japanese patients as they could not receive organs in their own country. Since the law's revision, however, these patients should have no need to seek transplants overseas, but numbers of donations from this age group have not increased, and only five cases of organ donations from brain-dead children have taken place (up to July 25, 2014). Thus, most child recipients—especially heart recipient candidates—are still either dependent on overseas transplants or waiting for organs in Japan.

THE PARTIALLY REVISED LAW (JANUARY 17, 2010 TO PRESENT)

Between the original Japanese organ transplantation law and its revision there was a partial change in the law on January 17, 2010, just six months before the main revision. The change was called the "family-first organ donor rule," through which Japanese people could carry a donor card that made their organs available for donation first to their family members. This rule received opposing reactions throughout the world, based on cultural differences: in the West it was considered unfair (against the fundamental principles of the "gift of life"), while in the Far East it was perceived as natural to wish to prioritize family members (everybody wants to save beloved family members). The rule also contained certain conditions for donor candidates.

1. *Donor Candidate Age Limit*

Under the "family-first organ donor rule," donor candidates must be over the age of fifteen years and must have their own signed donor card to donate to specific named family members. This age limit continued from the original Japanese organ transplantation law, despite the fact that the fully revised law six months later repealed the age limit to give children the opportunity to donate and receive organs. Nevertheless the limit remains in place for the "family-first organ donor rule," meaning that anyone aged fourteen and under is prohibited from donating their organs under this rule, even though the main organ transplantation law now allows it.

2. *Family Definition*

The rule states that "family" includes only spouses, children, and parents, who must be named as the organ recipients on the donor card. In the modern world, families are frequently more diverse than this definition would imply, including common-law married couples, as well as step-siblings and step-parents. The "family-first organ donor rule" doesn't take any of these other family relationships into account, which can cause sensitive issues for the donor candidate and the potential recipients.

3. *Medical Condition*

The rule also insists that donor candidates must meet the specific medical conditions required by each recipient. A typical medical problem encountered in transplantation is blood type mismatching: for example, a donation from a blood type A donor to a blood type A recipient or a blood type AB recipient is compatible, while a blood type B donor cannot donate to a blood type A recipient. When the donor and the donor's named recipient candidate are blood group incompatible, it is impossible to transplant an organ between them, even though they are within the same family circle.

This condition is the same as in ordinary organ donation under the main law, but it means that the list of candidates that must be checked for the organ to be donated may be longer than usual. However, the time limit on how quickly organs must be transplanted is very strict—for example, a maximum of four hours can elapse between a heart being harvested from a donor and transplanted to a recipient. Under the "family-first organ donor rule," if Donor A's donor card names Candidate B but they are a medical mismatch, Donor A's organ will be offered to another family member, Candidate C. If there is no matching family member, Donor A must donate the organ to a candidate outside the family circle.

This tracing of potential donors before donors on a hospital waiting list can be considered exhausts some of the available time before the transplant must take place.

4. Conditions for Donating

The rule is somewhat complex and also contains four conditions for being a donor to a named recipient. This section outlines the conditions and offers practical case examples to provide more specific details.

1. When a family recipient cannot accept the organ for medical reasons, the organ will be donated instead to a recipient outside the family who is a candidate on a waiting list. For example, a mother of two children with no other family tries to donate her kidney to her daughter, who is named on her donor card, but her kidney and her daughter's body (or their blood types) are a mismatch so it cannot be done. She may then try to donate to her son if he is also named on the donor card, but if they encounter another mismatch then she must donate to an unknown recipient candidate on a waiting list outside her family circle (she cannot refuse to donate others).

2. When a family member is named on a donor card, all family members can receive the donor's organs. For example, a mother tries to donate her kidney to her daughter, but they are a mismatch. Her donation is then available to her son if he needs it. If he is also a mismatch, her kidney becomes available to any other recipient candidates inside her family circle, not just those named on the donor card.

3. When a potential donor refuses organ donation except to the named family member, his/her donation will be inadmissible to all. For example, a mother tries to donate her kidney to her daughter, then other members of her family, but finds no matches. If she thereafter refuses to donate her kidney to an unknown recipient candidate outside her family circle on a waiting list, she loses any opportunity to become an organ donor. She is then forbidden to donate her organs not only to unknown recipients but also to family members who may need them in the future.

4. Suicides are not permitted to donate their organs, in order to avoid the possibility that donors might consider suicide in order to donate. For example, a mother decides to kill herself to try to donate her kidney to her daughter as quickly as possible. She thus loses any opportunity to become an organ donor, either to her daughter or any other recipient. Japanese assessments of suicide donors are in any case very negative, and recipients tend to avoid suicide donors because of an abhorrence of this type of death, which is

perceived as a bad omen. Nevertheless, there is evidence that some suicides and attempted suicides have donated organs in Japan already, and may be very keen to donate their organs.

The "family-first organ donor rule" was implemented on January 17, 2010, but did not initially work well; it seemed to have no impact on the population at all. However, after the organ transplantation law was revised completely on July 17, 2010, and family-presumed consent and the "family-first organ donor rule" were combined, this produced a much more advantageous effect. This result was far from predictable, but the phenomenon suggests that Japanese people prefer to rely on family-presumed consent, rather than insisting on individual organ donation wills. In addition, Japanese culture appears to favor organ donation within the family circle—an approach shared within the Far East—even though this attitude is perceived as unfair in the West. For Japanese people (and for other cultures in the Far East), donating organs to family members seems very natural, while donating to strangers is not.

This may stem in part from the religious mix in Japan, which combines traditional indigenous beliefs; Shinto, a polytheistic religion created in Japan more recently; Buddhism, which arrived in Japan via India and China in the sixth century; and Christianity, which was brought to Japan in 1549 (although less than 1 percent of the population is Christian). Many Japanese people combine these various beliefs in their daily lives—for example, holding a Shinto wedding, a Buddhist funeral, and celebrating Christmas in winter. This syncretization of many religions may stem less from piety and more from enjoyment of religious events. Since the fifth century most Japanese have also followed the ethics and philosophy of Confucianism, which is relatively common in the Far East, and in which mutilating the body (including even body piercing and surgery) is taboo—although this has lessened somewhat in recent years—but great stress is laid on taking care of the family circle above all others.

The development of Japanese organ transplantation law has followed a unique route as a result of the "Wada case," and the legal situation still causes significant problems in the field. The reasons behind the extremely slow advances in organ transplantation uptake in Japan are a combination of cultural and traditional mores and the nightmarish and scandalous "Wada case."

Bibliography

BOOKS AND ARTICLES

Abe, T. (1994). "Cultural Theory of Life." In *Why Is Brain-Dead Transplantation a Problem? Messages from Medical Doctors against the Brain-Dead Transplantation Law*, edited by Y. Watanabe and T. Abe. Tokyo: Yumiru Publisher, 219–221.

Arimura, H. (1999). *Not Received a Gift*. Tokyo: Keizaikai Co. Ltd.

Awaya, T. (2002). "Exploitation of Resources and Commercialization of Human Body and Modern Human Body Ownership." *Associé* 9, 101–112.

Benedict, R. (1946). *The Chrysanthemum and the Sword: Patterns of Japanese Culture*. Boston, MA: Houghton Mifflin.

Fox, R., and Swazey, J. (1992). *Spare Parts: Organ Replacement in American Society*. New York: Oxford University Press.

Inhorn, M., and Wentzell, E. (2011). "Embodying Emergent Masculinities: Reproductive and Sexual Health Technologies in the Middle East and Mexico." *American Ethnologist* 38(4), 801–815.

Kleinman, A. (1980). *Patients and Healers in the Context of Culture: An Exploration of the Borderland between Anthropology, Medicine, and Psychiatry*. Oakland: University of California Press.

———. (1988). *The Illness Narratives: Suffering, Healing and the Human Condition*. New York: Basic Books.

Koyama, K. (2009). *Okuribito* [*Departures*], original scenario. Tokyo: Shogakukan.

Kyodo News Service: Organ Transplant Group of Reporters of City News. (1998). *A Frozen Heart*. Tokyo: Kyodo News Service.

Lock, M. (2002). *Twice Dead: Organ Transplants and the Reinvention of Death*. Berkeley: University of California Press.

Mauss, M. (1954). *The Gift: Forms and Functions of Exchange in Archaic Societies*, translated by I. Cunnison. London: Cohen and West Ltd.

Namihira, E. (1996). *Cultural Anthropology of Life*. Tokyo: Shinchosha Co. Ltd.

Setoyama, M. (2001). '"My Recommended 10 Best Books for Students and Residents." *Medical Community Weekly World Newspaper* 16(4), 24–34.

Starzl, T. (1992). *The Puzzle People: Memories of a Transplant Surgeon*. Pittsburgh: University of Pittsburgh Press.

Todo, S. (2000). "Key People of the 21st Century." *Yomiuri Year Book 2000*. Tokyo: The Yomiuri Shimbun.

Uchimura, E. (2013). *Gendai Nohon no Sousou Bunka* [*Current Japanese Funeral Culture*]. Tokyo: Iwata-Shoin.

Yasuoka, M. K. (2004). "Six Patterns of Grieving Processes in Organ-Donating Decision Makers: Narratives from 5 Donor Families." *Challenges for Bioethics from Asia*, Eubios Ethics Institute, New Zealand, 274–281.

———. (2006). "Rebirthable Life: Medical Anthropology Study of the Concept of Life According to Concerned Parties Involved in Brain Death and Organ Transplantation." PhD thesis: Department of History and Anthropology (Medical Anthropology), Graduate School of Letters, Hokkaido University, Sapporo, Japan (unpublished).

———. (2010). "Medical Refugees in Japan: From Overseas Transplants to Organ Self-Sufficiency for Japanese Recipients." *Applied Ethics: Challenges for the 21st Century.*

Sapporo, Japan: Center for Applied Ethics and Philosophy, Hokkaido University, 85–97.

———— (2011). "Revision of Organ Transplantation Law in Japan: Brain Death, Presumed Consent, and Donation of Children's Organs." In Center for Applied Ethics and Philosophy, *Applied Ethics: Old Wine in New Bottles?* Sapporo, Japan: Center for Applied Ethics and Philosophy, Hokkaido University, 186–198.

————. (2013). "Rebirthable Life: Narratives and Reproductive Life of Japanese Brain-Dead Donors." *Research Journal of Graduate Students of Letters* (Japan) 8, 73–81.

WEB PAGES

American Society of Transplantation, http://www.myast.org/ (home page), accessed 05/05/2014.

American Society of Transplant Surgeons, http://www.asts.org/ (home page), accessed 05/05/2014.

Aoyagi Ceremonial Hall, http://www.ch-aoyagi.co.jp/index.html (home page), accessed 10/11/2014.

Eubios Ethics Institute, http://www.biol.tsukuba.ac.jp/~macer/index.html (home page), accessed 05/05/2014.

EUROTRANSPLANT, http://www.eurotransplant.org/cms/ (home page), accessed 05/05/2014

HRSA (US Department of Health and Human Services, Health Resources and Services Administration), http://www.hrsa.gov/ (home page), accessed 05/05/2014.

Japan Organ Transplant Network, http://www.jotnw.or.jp/english/01.html (The history of transplanting), accessed 09/30/2014.

Japan Transplant Recipients Organization, http://www.jtr.ne.jp/index.html (home-page), accessed 09/16/2014.

Jikenshi Tankyu [Criminal Case Histories], http://jikenshi.web.fc2.com/newpage201. htm (Wada case), accessed 05/12/2014.

LifeLink—The Organ Donation Network http://www.organ.redcross.org.au/ (home page), accessed 05/09/2014.

Medical Information Network Society, http://www.medi-net.or.jp/tcnet/index_e.html (Transplant communication) accessed 04/17/2014.

Ministry of Health, Labor and Welfare, http://www.mhlw.go.jp/english/ (home page), accessed 05/05/2014.

NHSBT (National Health Service Blood and Transplant), http://www.nhsbt.nhs.uk/ (home page), accessed 05/05/2014.

Organ Watch, http://sunsite3.berkeley.edu/biotech/organwatch/ (home page), accessed 05/09/2014.

Project Bionics, http://echo.gmu.edu/bionics (Artificial organs from discovery to clinical use: an ASAIO history project at The Smithsonian), accessed 04/17/2014).

The Australian Heart Lung Transplant Association (AHLTA), http://www.ahlta.com/ (home page), accessed 05/09/2014.

The Declaration of Istanbul on Organ Trafficking and Transplant Tourism, http://www.declarationofistanbul.org/ (home page), accessed 05/05/2014.

The Transplantation Society, http://www.tts.org/ (home page), accessed 05/05/2014.

Trans Web, http://www.transweb.org/ (home page), accessed 05/09/2014.

United Network for Organ Sharing (UNOS), http://www.unos.org/ (home page), accessed 05/05/2014.

World Health Organization (WHO), http://www.who.int/en/ (home page), accessed 05/05/2014.

Index

organ donations, 49–50, 169; attitudes
  to, 72–74; conditions for, 173–174;
  for donor families, 68–69; of
  kidneys, 50, 65n2, 173; narratives of,
  93–96; overseas, 53; rates, 10, 11, 12,
  32, 44, 47, 54–55, 168–169, 169
organ harvesting: bioethics as against,
  117; overview of, 23–26; for
  recipients, 28–29; for recipients'
  families, 29–30; surgeons'
  motivation for, 11
organ mediators: donor and, 109; at
  Transplant Games, 110
organ reception, 43; agreeing to, 45–47;
  attitudes to, 50–53, 63; narratives of,
  91–93; reasons for, 45–47; in
  recipient narratives, 50–53;
  recipients' reactions to, 44–45, 63
organ recipients. *See* recipients
organ rejection, 49–50. *See also*
  cyclosporine
organ replacement. *See* transplantation
organs: as artificial, 5–6; biological life
  received from, 111; body
  replacement of, 127–128; at
  hospitals, 11; as living, 121; shelf life
  of, 131; shortage, 6, 24, 44, 48, 50,
  54–55, 68, 129, 168–169, 169;
  survival of, 107; in thank you letter,
  107; trafficking in, 168, 171. *See also*
  rebirthable life
organ self-sufficiency, 8, 47, 168, 171
organ tourism, 8, 10
organ tracking, 8
"Organ Transplantation" (Yamauchi),
  6
Osaka, Japan, 124
Oseibo, 54, 118–119
"other", 151
overseas donations, from brain-dead
  donors, 53
overseas surgery, 8, 10, 48, 65n1, 65n2,
  92–93; in Australia, 56–58; children
  dependent on, 171; in U.S., 59–60,
  62, 97, 102

pancreas specialist. *See* Toyota
pancreas transplant. *See* Satoshi
parents, 46

partially revised law, 171–174
part-time workers, 78, 83
patients: dead people saving, 130;
  doctor's relationship with, 91; gift
  of, 123; informed consent given up
  on by, 21, 46; in overseas surgery,
  48; surgeon's relationship with,
  45–46; as unconscious, 164–165
patriarchy, 75–76
pediatrician, 46
personal donation will, 74
philosophies, 40
physician narratives: gift of life in, 32;
  quitting in, 31, 32; recipients in, 31.
  See also Matsui
pillow service (*makura-gyo*), 158, 159
praying, 125–126
pride, in renewable life, 133
privacy, of donor families, 68
promotion, 126
pulling friends (*tomobiki*), 158
The Puzzle People (Starzl), 123

quitting, in physician narratives, 31, 32

Raia, Silvano, 7
rebirthable life, 87–88, 118; advocacy
  caused by, 140; concerned parties
  influenced by, 135–136, 147–151,
  152; daughter in, 142; death in, 140;
  decision in, 139; by donor families,
  141–144, 144; as dramatic, 137;
  enchantment in, 138; feelings in,
  140–141; generosity in, 143; healing
  in, 143; husband in, 143; love in,
  136–137; medical technologies
  giving, 151; overview of, 135–136,
  144, 145, 147–151, 152; partial save
  in, 138; by recipients, 139–141, 144;
  son in, 141–142, 142–143;
  supernatural power in, 137–138; by
  surgeons, 136–138, 144; treasure in,
  137
recipient coordinators, 11, 23, 25, 40;
  dilemmas of, 26–27, 28, 28–30;
  narratives, 37–38, 39. *See also* Morita;
  Toyota
recipient narratives, 49–50; advocacy
  in, 51; children in, 46, 49; death in,

About the Author

Maria-Keiko Yasuoka is visiting researcher at the Hokkaido University School of Medicine in Japan. Her work focuses on anthropological and bioethical aspects of emerging medical technologies such as organ transplantation.